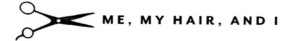

**ME, MY HAIR, AND I**

. . . . . . . . . . . . . . . . . . . . . . . .

# ME,
# MY HAIR,
# AND I

. . . . . . . . . . . . . . . . . . . . . . . .

*Edited by*

## ELIZABETH BENEDICT

ALGONQUIN BOOKS OF CHAPEL HILL   2015

Published by

ALGONQUIN BOOKS OF CHAPEL HILL
Post Office Box 2225
Chapel Hill, North Carolina 27515-2225

a division of
WORKMAN PUBLISHING
225 Varick Street
New York, New York 10014

Library of Congress Cataloging-in-Publication Data
Me, my hair, and I : twenty-seven women untangle an obsession /
edited by Elizabeth Benedict.—1st ed.
pages cm
ISBN 978-1-61620-814-1
1. Hair. 2. Hair—Social aspects. 3. Hairstyles—Social aspects.
4. Women—Identity. 5. Women—Health and hygiene. 6. Women
authors—United States. I. Benedict, Elizabeth.
GT2290.M4 2015
646.7'24—dc23                                     2015011132

10 9 8 7 6 5 4 3 2 1
First Edition

*For Nancy, James, Emily, and Julia*

"To be born woman is to know—
Although they do not talk of it at school—
That we must labour to be beautiful."
—w. b. yeats, "Adam's Curse"


Wouldn't they be surprised when one day I woke out of my black ugly dream, and my real hair, which was long and blond, would take the place of the kinky mass that Momma wouldn't let me straighten?
—maya angelou, *I Know Why the Caged Bird Sings*


It's like the medical field. Aside from people being born and dying, women will spend their last dime to get their hair done, so I'll always have a job.
—sahara, a student at the Beauty Schools of America, Miami Beach, Florida, on why she's chosen to be a hairstylist

# CONTENTS

· · · · · · · · · · · · · · · · · · · · · · ·

## ACKNOWLEDGMENTS

. . . . . . . . . . . . . . . . . . . . . . .

As always, I am indebted to Gail Hochman and Marianne Merola for their steady, serious devotion to the work of fostering authors and books, in this case my own. Andra Miller is a writer's dream of an editor, and Algonquin a writer's dream of a publisher. I offer my heartfelt gratitude to everyone there who has worked on *What My Mother Gave Me* and *Me, My Hair, and I.* Outside the publishing world, I want to acknowledge Thea Piltzecker, who put me in touch with one of the contributors.

It's impossible to sufficiently thank the writers who've shared their deepest feelings about their families, their spouses, their children, their cultures, their religions, their illnesses, and, oh, yes, their hair! in these scintillating essays. I hope this is just the start of a long public conversation about what we all talk about when we talk about hair—because we talk about *everything:* politics, passion, motherhood, mortality, vanity, self-doubt, self-loathing, self-esteem, rebirth, regeneration, and, occasionally, the deep pleasure of a really great haircut.

Hairwise and otherwise, I'm grateful to my sister, Nancy Neiditz, who once delivered a comic lecture at a posh New York restaurant—pointing out women around the dining room—on the immutable desirability of straight hair, which had everyone at our table doubled over in laughter, especially those with curly hair. Her devotion to her own hair puts me to shame. I'm immensely grateful for the company and inspiration of my niece Julia Smith, who wears her hair very short and no longer bright green; to my stepdaughter, Emily Daggett Smith, who wears her long hair with style and elegance; and to my husband, James Smith, who puts up with my tangled, sometimes Phyllis Diller–like tresses with great good humor. Best of all, on those occasions when I get my hair done, he notices.

# INTRODUCTION

ASK A WOMAN about her hair, and she just might tell you the story of her life.

Ask a whole bunch of women, and if *Me, My Hair, and I* is any indication, you could get a history of the world: reflections and revelations about family, race, religion, ritual, culture, politics, celebrity, what goes on in African American kitchens and at Hindu Bengali weddings in Calcutta, alongside stories about the influence of Jackie Kennedy, Angela Davis, Lena Horne, Madonna, Audrey Hepburn, Shirley Temple, Sandra Dee, Joan Baez, Farrah Fawcett, Kelly McGillis, Judith Butler, the Grateful Dead, and Botticelli's Venus.

What's abundantly clear in all these personal stories is that hair matters. Many other facts of life matter too, oftentimes more than hair (illness, poverty, war, famine, flood, and sometimes shoes and makeup), but hair can be counted on to matter just about every day, at least to a high percentage of women—and to more than a few men, at least back in the day. The Beatles' long hair, when it first shimmied and shook on

*The Ed Sullivan Show* in 1964, in time to "I Want to Hold Your Hand," changed the course of social history. Way before that, the Old Testament's Samson believed that his hair, seven braids' worth, was the source of his strength, and his enemies hired the temptress Delilah to cut if off.

As I read and reflect on these essays, I'm struck by just how much hair matters to so many of us, and by the tangled intricacies of why. Why so much? And why with this intensity?

"A woman's hair is her glory," Maya Angelou explains in *Good Hair*, Chris Rock's documentary about African American women and their hair. But long before it has a chance to acquire glory in our lives, it demands attention and care. It's an early life lesson in basic grooming, a public window into the private household. In social science terms, hair is a signifier. One of the earliest signals it transmits, when we're kids, is whether we are being looked after properly. A child's unkempt hair invites scrutiny, condemnation, and, if it's really a mess day after day, maybe a visit from Child Protective Services. As girls grow up and learn to groom their own hair, they learn to take care of themselves. When they have daughters, they groom them too, and so the cycle continues. Along the way, we learn that the hair choices we make for ourselves and others reveal who we are, the worlds we live in, and how we want to be perceived.

For women, hair is an entire library of information, about status, class, self-image, desire, sexuality, values, and even mental health. For many of the years I lived in Washington, DC, in the 1980s, I remember frequently seeing a woman with gnarled, matted hair that stood a foot off her scalp. She was protesting—I think it was nuclear war—on the sidewalk outside the White House. While I shared her views on nuclear war, the state of her hair told me that she was not entirely well. I can summon her face vividly, but I know the reason I always noticed her was the house of hair atop her head.

Hair matters because it's always *around*, framing our faces, growing in, falling out, getting frizzy, changing colors—in short, demanding our attention: Comb me! Wash me! Relax me! Color me! It's always *there*, conveying messages about who we are and what we want. Invite me to the prom! Love me! Hire me! Sleep with me! Don't even think about sleeping with me! Take me seriously! Marry me! Mistake me—please!—for a much-younger woman!

It's always there, unless it's gone or it's hidden—and those absences tell stories too. A common one involves the ravages of chemotherapy; missing hair is evidence of illness. Then there are cultures where women shave off their hair and cover their heads, and other cultures where women may keep their hair, but their heads must be shrouded in veils, sometimes with only slits or screens through which to see. Why the shaved heads? Why the draperies? There are many reasons and many interpretations, depending on one's relationship to the veils. Covering the hair signifies membership, to insiders and outsiders, in a specific group; it's a quick self-identifier. It may remind members of the group how to worship and to behave. It focuses attention on the face, not the secondary characteristics. And shaving or hiding the hair fundamentally nullifies hair's ornamental, aesthetic, and sexual properties, thereby sending unambiguous messages about the women's availability and independence. Finally, there's the hair that's almost always hidden from view—but that has crept into public conversations in the past two decades, as Brazilian waxes, dyes, bleaches, and other grooming gimmicks have made achieving childlike genitals the new normal.

Not surprisingly, there seems to be a hair story in the news just about every day, and because we live in the twenty-first century, most of these stories then leap to Twitter, Facebook, and TMZ, and heavens knows where else. Before long, the whole world—or just a few thousand people—is debating Jennifer Aniston's layers, Michelle Obama's bangs, the toxins in hair dyes, the Duchess of Cambridge's teasing her husband about his bald spot, a movie star on a TMI jag about her pubic hair, a child expelled from school for a hairstyle, an Olympic gymnast condemned for her kinky hair, and the US Army's issuing new rules about which hairstyles are permitted and which are not.

News stories about hair run the gamut from pop-culture fluff to ethnic and racial hot buttons, and the hottest of those often involve African Americans and their tresses. If we're black, we know the landscape of this territory intimately. If we're not, we may be oblivious to the very separate world of African American hair, an issue so complex and charged that it's been the subject of dozens of books—histories, self-help, and photo essays. Long before *Good Hair*, Maya Angelou told her own hair history in *I Know Why the Caged Bird Sings*, and in his autobiography, Malcolm X describes his introduction to getting his hair straightened into a "conk," using lye, eggs, and potatoes, and later his condemnation of this brutal technique.

In African American culture, "good hair" is smooth and soft. For many of the other contributors, "good hair" is also the straight hair that they don't have naturally and always wanted. As all unhappy families are different in their own ways, each story here of a woman at war with her hair is unique. Fortunately, not all contributors have had such adversarial relationships, though family conflict and connection were often acted out through the writers' hair and the locks of other family members.

While it's easy to make light of our obsession with our hair, very few of the writers in these pages do that. We get that hair is serious. It's our glory, our nemesis, our history, our sexuality, our religion, our vanity, our joy, and our mortality. It's true that there are many things in life that matter more than hair, but few that matter in quite these complicated, energizing, and interconnected ways. As near as I can tell, that's the long and short of it.

ME, MY HAIR, AND I

# The Rapunzel Complex

REBECCA NEWBERGER GOLDSTEIN

I'VE NEVER FIGURED OUT how to tell the story of my life. But I do think I can tell the story of my hair.

My hair grew up in the shadow of my older sister's hair, which was long and golden and spilled in beautiful natural curls onto her shoulders. My hair was also light but always described as dirty blond, which led to confusion. I was never able to get across to my mother why she so often found me in the upstairs bathroom, taking a bar of Ivory soap to my hair and scrubbing. If I'd belonged to a different kind of family, neuroses might have been suspected and I might have been taken to a therapist.

Even more than clean hair, I wanted long hair. But my mother was tired by the time my younger sister and I were born. There were twelve years between the oldest of my siblings and the youngest; I was born after a large gap. It was as if there were two different sets, the older children my mother took pleasure in and then the pair of us, Sarah and I, both with short hair. I must really have wanted long hair to have raised the issue with my mother at all. She was short tempered when she responded that my hair was too thick to be grown long. Untangling it would only add to the burdens of her life. In my mind, my hair's thickness was connected with its dirtiness, making the contrast between my older sister's tresses of glory and my own ugly hair even greater. My mother cut my too-thick locks, and since she didn't want to have to do it often, my hair was cut very short, shorter even than Sarah's. The last part of the ordeal was my father's running his electric shaver over the back of my neck to clean away the stubble. I hated the pinching feel of that electric shaver, and I hated my boy cuts.

As soon as I gained autonomy over my own head, I grew my hair with utter abandon. In college it was so long that I could sit on it. Sarah also grew her hair long, and this being the late sixties, we took turns ironing each other's tresses to suppress any bourgeois pro-war tendencies toward curling. One day when I was lying with my head in the hands of my sister, I heard her say in a frightened voice, "Something's gone wrong." The stench reached me almost simultaneously with Sarah's words. She'd neglected to turn down the heat setting. A wad of scorched hair was melded to the reeking iron. Once again, I had to cut my hair short, but by the time I got my PhD, it was hippie-long again.

When I got my first job teaching philosophy, I was twenty-six and looked far younger. The students always seemed a bit confused the first day of class when I strode to the front of the room to take command. Their skepticism intensified my own sense of absurdity at having my words dutifully written down by smart Barnard women. Who was I to be accorded such status? Perhaps a sophisticated haircut would convince us all of my authority. I asked around and was given the name of the salon said to be the best in Manhattan. Kenneth, I was told, had created Jacqueline Kennedy's bouffant hairdo. I took my hair to Kenneth's, and though I didn't receive the attentions of the celebrity hairdresser himself, still I could tell this was a dauntingly classy establishment. I had overreached myself in trying to do justice to my hair and was unprepared to resist the professional argument, authoritatively delivered, to the effect that my hair must, simply *must*, be cut far shorter than I'd anticipated. I watched it pile up on the floor, afraid to raise my eyes to the mirror. When I finally did, the look on my face prompted the

*Being the late sixties, we took turns ironing each other's tresses to suppress any bourgeois pro-war tendencies toward curling.*

hairdresser to ask me whether "philosophy majors" ever cry. Damn it, I wanted to tell him. I'm not a philosophy major. I'm a philosophy professor! A professor! That's the only reason I'm sitting here with all my hair lying detached from my head only to become garbage on your pricey floor!

Since that learning experience at Kenneth's, I have tried never to betray my hair. As a child I already knew that I possessed long hair that was trapped inside a short cut. I also figured out, as I got older, that I was a freethinker trapped within Orthodox Judaism, a feminist trapped in paternalism, a novelist trapped in the rules of my own rigorous academic discipline. My hair's struggles have been my struggles.

*As a child I already knew that I possessed long hair that was trapped inside a short cut.*

I kept it long, but there were still mistakes to be made along the way. A hairdresser once made the argument that at my age—I had just turned forty—women look better, which is to say younger, as redheads. As a philosopher I'm trained to spot the fallacies in arguments, but somehow I was duped by this one. I was going to have to see this hairdresser every eight weeks in order for my roots to be attended to. By about the third session, I caught on and went back to my natural color. I was buried under obligations. Not only did I teach now, but I was writing novels. And I had two daughters, both of whom had long, long hair. I didn't have time for hair salon appointments every eight weeks. And anyway, I wasn't any redhead.

My children brought their own pressures to bear on my hair. At around the age of ten, my older daughter became acutely embarrassed by the look I had evolved. I looked nothing like the other mothers in our suburban New Jersey community. She begged me to never wear my army boots when I picked her up from school, and this being the eighties, she begged me to get a perm. I remembered my own acute embarrassment prompted by my own mother, who, as an Orthodox woman, looked nothing like the chic women of White Plains, New York, where I'd grown up. All of them were slim and tall and tanned. They seemed to have tennis rackets growing out of their hands, where my mother had a spatula (which I believed to be a Yiddish word). And so, remembering, I took my daughter's embarrassment to heart. It took about six months for that awful perm to grow out.

Her younger sister, a nonconformist from an early age, complained about my looks only once. I'd come to pick her up at the end of her summer program, run each year by Johns Hopkins University. My marriage had recently broken up, and I'd decided to update my look. I was wearing a stylish sleeveless black dress, and I'd added highlights to my hair that had finally lifted it out of the category of dirty blond. My daughter took one look at me and said, in the perfected disdain of her fifteen years, "Now you look just like all the other mothers of the preppies up here. Are you in training to become a trophy wife?" She was in a mood to draw blood, which I acknowledged and respected, but still I couldn't help bursting out in laughter. I'd just turned fifty. Some trophy.

The beautiful golden hair of my older sister had gone through its own life story. She'd remained Orthodox, and in her circle she was supposed to wear a wig, or at least to keep her hair covered beneath a kerchief or a hat. But Mynda had resisted. Her hair had always been her glory. She resisted death with the same spirit. Lying in the hospital only days before the end, she asked me to comb her hair. Although it had pitifully thinned, it was still there, lying spread out on her shoulders; and this itself seemed a triumph. We joked that vanity would be the last thing in either of us to go. My beautiful sister.

*My hair and I have grown into ourselves and know what we're about.*

My hair has partaken in the high points of my life. A reviewer in the *London Times* once referred to me as "the American philosopher-novelist who looks like Rapunzel but thinks like Wittgenstein." That was nice. And when I was inducted into the American Academy of Arts and Sciences, I was seated next to the novelist Alison Lurie. At the close of the ceremony my partner, Steven Pinker, approached us, and

I pointed him out to Alison. She gave him a long, appraising look. "Good hair" was her verdict. Then she gave me the same once-over. "You too," she said. "You're the good-hair couple," she pronounced. Worse things have been said about both of us.

My hair is still long, no doubt inappropriately so for my age, but I am perhaps also of an age when no one dares—or cares—to say such a thing to me anymore. I've kept the highlights too, and they mask the gray that comes in around the temples during the long stretches in between my salon visits. Nobody will ever convince me again to do anything with my hair but what I want. My hair and I have grown into ourselves and know what we're about.

The only one who ever has any hair suggestion to make is Steve. When I tell him that I'm off to the salon for one of my rare trims, he never fails to admonish, "Don't let them cut too much off. I love your hair long." Which, for the story of my hair, and now his, is another way of saying, And they lived happily ever after.

# Hair, Interrupted

SULEIKA JAOUAD

**F**OR AS LONG as I can remember I've felt like an outsider looking in. Between the ages of four and eighteen, I attended six schools on three continents. As the child of two immigrants—my mother is Swiss and my father is Tunisian—I discovered that my multicultural background was anything but "cool" or "exotic" to my classmates. Roll call on the first day of school was like showing up to class wearing underwear on the outside of my jeans. With a name as unpronounceable as Suleika Jaouad, I found it hard to blend in. Sometimes that made me want to blend in all the more.

Even my lunch box was a source of embarrassment. All I wanted back then was a brown paper bag filled with typical, all-American fare: peanut butter and jelly sandwiches, Snackables,

Pop-Tarts, and Gushers. Was that too much to ask for? I remember bursting through the door after school in a huff one day. "Never, *ever* pack me chicken tagine for lunch again," I said. The contrast between the smelly, coagulated orange mess of chicken and the pristine, odorless beauty of a Pop-Tart had never felt sharper.

Over time, the embarrassment of being the perpetual new kid hardened into resentment. I resented that my family had a French-only language policy at home. I resented that I had a multisyllabic name and that I was too young to legally change it to something more normal like Ashley or Jessica. And I resented that my mother, an artist with a flair for the eccentric and a sturdy sense of who she was and what she believed, seemed to think it was so easy to be comfortable with not always fitting in. "You are unique," she would tell me, forgetting that the word is a social albatross when you're a kid. I was mortified the day she came to pick me up at the bus stop wearing cross-country skis, a fluorescent-yellow parka, and a backward baseball cap covering her spiky two-inch-long hairdo. *Quelle horreur!*

When I got to middle school and my family settled in upstate New York, I dreamed of having golden, waist-length Rapunzel-like tresses—like the popular girls on the cheerleading squad—instead of my frizzy, shoulder-length auburn hair. I tried everything. They knew me in the hair product aisle at the local CVS pharmacy, but no amount of roasting my hair with Sun-In or dousing it in Long 'N Strong could make me look like *them*. In the sixth grade, I even persuaded my mother to let me get a braided blond weave (hello, fashion police!).

These were the memories that came rushing back to me on a muggy spring afternoon in May 2011, at the age of twenty-two. Nothing of note was happening in the news that day. But the world that I knew was about to implode.

"Precautionary" was the word the doctor had used. He was talking about the bone marrow biopsy I had undergone a few days before, a fairly painful, invasive procedure that is rarely performed on young people. After two months of flu-like symptoms that seemed resistant to the strongest antibiotics, it had been the next step. My skin had become so pale it looked almost translucent. "Robin's egg blue, as if all of the veins have floated to the surface of my skin," was how I described it in my journal. Something was wrong. This much I knew. But the doctor reassured me that he didn't expect to find anything abnormal in my bone marrow.

By the time my parents and I arrived at the clinic to hear the results of the biopsy, it was dusk. All of the staff and the other patients had gone for the day. The lights in the waiting room had been dimmed, casting an ominous shadow on the beige walls and stacks of outdated magazines. The doctor didn't mince words. "You have something called acute myeloid leukemia," he said, enunciating the diagnosis like a foreign-language teacher instructing us in the pronunciation of a new vocabulary word. "We need to act fast."

*Chemotherapy is a take-no-prisoners stylist.*

A lot of people have asked me what it was like to hear that I had cancer at such a young age. What's the appropriate reaction to one's own cancer diagnosis? Are you supposed to break down in tears, or faint, or scream?

I did not do any of those things. Instead, I froze and repeated the word over and over in my head: *Loo-kee-mee-ah. Loo-kee-mee-ah. Loo-kee-mee-ah.* It sounded like an exotic flower.

It was my next reaction, however, that really surprised me. "Am I going to lose all my hair?" I blurted out to the doctor.

On balance, since I had just been diagnosed with a life-threatening illness, worrying about hair loss seemed petty and irrelevant, even narcissistic. But a bald head—the signature side effect of chemotherapy—was one of the few tropes that I knew about cancer. I needed to reassure myself by asking questions that were within the realm of my understanding. A question like, What's going to happen to me? could have lethal and terrifyingly unforeseeable consequences. My doctor confirmed that the chemo would take my hair as its prize, within a week or so of starting treatment.

CHEMOTHERAPY IS A take-no-prisoners stylist. The thing that no one tells you when you lose your hair during chemo is that it doesn't happen all at once. The first evidence that mine was falling out appeared on my pillow: a mess of stray hairs spread across the fabric like a furry Jackson Pollock painting. Then, over the next few days, it started to come out in clumps. Finally, when only a few patches of hair were left on my head, I yanked the rest of it out with my bare hands. I felt like a gardener, pulling weeds from damp soil.

Within a few weeks, I could no longer recognize the person staring back at me in the mirror. Gaunt cheeks. Bald head. No eyebrows. No eyelashes. Skin as dry and white as chalk. And a waist that quickly shrank from a healthy size 6 to a 00. But what hurt most were the silent, invisible side effects of my disease. The isolation. The friends who stopped returning my calls after I got sick. The fear of dying before I had really begun to live my life. And perhaps worst of all, coming to terms with the reality that the chemotherapy had rendered me permanently infertile. Just like that, my life had split in two: there was Suleika BC (before cancer) and Suleika AC (after cancer)—and that's if luck was on my side.

For the most part, my transformation had taken place within the privacy of the four walls of my hospital room. I could avoid the mirror hanging on the bathroom wall, but when I left the hospital for short breaks in between treatments, I couldn't shield myself from the stares of curious strangers. Everywhere

I went, cancer spoke for me before I could speak for myself. I tried hiding beneath hats and head scarves and wigs, but they only made me feel like more of an impostor.

One night, I made the mistake of going to a friend's party. It was my first time seeing many of my old college friends since my diagnosis. As I walked through the door, it felt like the music had suddenly gone dead. I could feel everyone's eyes glued to my bald head and to the tubes of my catheter protruding above my right breast. When I made eye contact with people, some quickly looked away. Conversations were awkward as acquaintances stared at their shoes or quickly excused themselves to make another drink or to go to the bathroom. A few minutes later, I told my friends I needed some fresh air. I jumped into a cab, hot, inky tears streaming down my face as I gave the driver directions to take me home.

*I was angry at the teenage version of myself, for nitpicking over the color and texture of my hair, when now I had no hair at all.*

My mom sat on the edge of my bed rubbing my back with the palms of her hands as I cried myself to sleep that night. I wanted my old life back, and I missed the way I had looked before. While my new situation was entirely unfamiliar territory for me, the feeling of wishing that I were in a different body—that I looked more similar to those around me—harked back to the way I had felt about myself in middle school. Now, however, I had a different perspective on the "outsider complex" of my youth. I was angry at the teenage version of myself, for nitpicking over the color and texture of my hair, when now I had no hair at all.

ALMOST A YEAR after my diagnosis, with three inches of freshly grown baby hair covering my head, I prepared for the most difficult chapter of my cancer treatment yet: a risky bone marrow transplant that would be my only shot at a cure. My doctors told me point-blank that I had a 35 percent chance of surviving the procedure. The odds were stacked against me. Surrounded by so much uncertainty, I began to search for the things that I *could* control. I realized that the outward signifiers of cancer could only define me if I allowed them to. I became determined to enter the transplant unit looking and feeling like Suleika, and not just an anonymous cancer patient.

Growing up, I had always wanted to wear the coveted cheerleader uniform. To be a girly girl. But I didn't want that anymore. I needed to look inward and to figure out what my own uniform was going to be. I adopted a brown leather jacket lent to me by my best friend, Lizzie. Boots with spikes on the heel staring at me in the store window? I'll take them. The final piece of my new look fell into place just five days before I was scheduled to enter the bone marrow transplant unit. I went to Astor Place Hairstylists, a cavernous basement barbershop in downtown Manhattan, known for its famously low prices, multilingual barbers, star-studded clientele, and no-nonsense customer service. I wanted to get a simple buzz cut, a pre-emptive strike against the chemo that would soon make my hair fall out for a second time.

When I explained my situation to my barber, Miguel Lora, he suggested I take the buzz cut one step further by getting "hair tattoos." The idea of a tattoo scared me at first, but Miguel reassured me that he would simply use his clippers to groove a spiral design in the half-inch layer of hair that remained. "What the hell," I said. After all, I had little left to lose. My new style made me look like I was tough, even when I didn't always feel that way. I was adding armor, and I liked the way it fit.

*My new style made me look like I was tough, even when I didn't always feel that way. I was adding armor, and I liked the way it fit.*

As I walked out onto the street, a construction worker whistled at me. "Cool hair!" he shouted out. It was the first time since my diagnosis that someone had made a remark on my appearance that wasn't cancer related.

WHILE CANCER MAY not be a choice, both style and attitude are. I wish I could have told this to my fifteen-year-old self. Trying to make my unruly brown locks blond back then was as futile an effort as trying to pretend that I had hair after my chemotherapy. I would never go so far as to call cancer a gift. After all, I would never give it to you for your birthday. But I would call it a teacher. My disease has taught me that I can far more effectively take control of my look by embracing it and having fun with it, rather than forcibly trying to make it something it is not. This approach toward my outward appearance extends into a larger lesson: no matter what life hurls your way, the best way to face a challenge is to lean into it and to make it your own.

Eventually, my hair would slowly start to grow back. As soon as it was long enough, I went to see Miguel for more hair tattoos. I shared photographs of my new hairstyle on social media, and within a few months, several other young cancer patients had gone to see Miguel to get their own hair tattoos. The tattoos had shown us a new way to have fun with the hair that we had—or that we didn't have—and given us a newfound confidence in our own skin.

I survived the bone marrow transplant. With each day, I'm getting stronger and healthier. And in the time since then, I've come to appreciate the benefits of sticking out in a crowd, even though I don't always seek out the circumstances. Today my hair is about two inches long, short and spiky just like my mother's. When people tell me how much we look alike, I smile and thank them for the compliment. I'm still a long way from having waist-length Rapunzel tresses. But the funny thing is, I don't want them anymore. Short hair is starting to grow on me.

# My Black Hair

. . . . . . . . . . . . . . . . . . . . . . . . . . . . . . . . . . . . . . . . . . . . . . . . . .

MARITA GOLDEN

If you are a Black woman, hair is serious business. Your hair is considered by many the definitive statement about who you are, who you think you are, and who you want to be. Long, thick, straight hair has for generations been considered a down payment on the American Dream. "Nappy" hair, although now accepted in its myriad forms, from the natural to twists and locks, has long been and remains a kind of bounced check on the acquisition of benefits of that same enduring cultural mythology. Like everything else about Black folk, Black people's—and especially Black women's—hair is knotted and gnarled by issues of race, politics, history, and pride.

Who would think that the family kitchen would double as a torture chamber? We think of the kitchen as the locus of nourishment, satisfaction, and family good times. But for generations of young Black girls, the family kitchen was associated with pain and fear, tears and dread. The kitchen was where, as a young girl, I got my hair "straightened." My coarse, sometimes called "kinky" or "nappy," hair, which was considered "bad" hair, got straightened with an iron comb that had been heated over a burner on the stove. It was made straight, as in no longer coarse, crooked, or "bad." Straight, as in the admonition I often heard shouted at children who were misbehaving, "Straighten yourself out." Ironically, "the kitchen" was also the name for the patch of unruly hair at the nape of the neck that was often most resistant to the magic of the hot comb.

> *If you are a Black woman, hair is serious business.*

Our kitchen in Washington, DC, smelled of smoke, burned hair, and Dixie Peach hair pomade, applied with my mother's fingers onto my scalp. Sometimes the "hot comb" was dipped into the hair pomade and then applied to my hair. My mother, like so many mothers, thought this was an art or a science, but in reality it was haphazard, even dangerous work when performed by amateurs. The result of this laborious and often, for me, degrading ritual was straight hair but burned ears, neckline, forehead, and scalp—all in the quest for what we called then, and many still call, "good hair."

I remember hating the every-two-week ordeal, or sometimes even more often, if a "touch-up" was required. Maybe my hair got wet in the rain, maybe I sweated too much playing outside, maybe, God forbid, I went swimming without a swim cap, and then we were back to square one. Back to that awful, horrible place where my hair was on my head in its natural state, not hurting me or anybody else, but coarse, tightly curled, and, to the eyes of so many around me, unacceptable. The process of losing the straightness of the hot comb was even called "going back." I got the message early on. I was not to face the world until my hair looked as near as it could to "good hair," also known as "White girl's hair." Is it any wonder that I soon developed the habit of standing in front of my mother's gilt-edged mirror with her silk scarves pinned on my head and imagining that those scarves were my real hair and that I had been transformed into Cinderella *and* Snow White? I spent count-

*Long, thick, straight hair has for generations been considered a down payment on the American Dream.*

less hours alone in front of that mirror, hypnotized by what I wished for and what my imagination had made real. To have a White girl's hair.

What happened to me in my mother's kitchen was part of the generations-old tradition and requirement in the Black community. For women and men to be accepted by and successful in both the Black and the White worlds, we had to look, either through hair texture, skin color, or phenotype, like Whites. Of the three, hair texture has always been the easiest to change.

Today, as Black women in America spend half a trillion dollars a year on weaves, wigs, braids, and relaxers, that 1950s fantasy lives on for new generations of Black women, who can now simply, easily, and cheaply buy what I wished for back then. Little Black girls still get the message that their hair needs to be tamed, but they don't wince and shrink as the hot comb nears their heads. As early as four or five years old, they are forced to endure "relaxers," a process in which harsh chemicals applied to their natural hair do what the hot comb did for me. And their tender young hair may not be strong enough yet to endure chemicals that are toxic and that with years-long use have raised questions about long-term health effects. Or long artificial extensions are braided into their natural hair, sometimes so tightly that scalp damage can occur.

*Black women's hair is knotted and gnarled by issues of race, politics, history, and pride.*

At about the age of twelve, I graduated from our kitchen to the beauty parlor on Fourteenth Street, where there were grown women in white uniforms—the professionals—who washed my hair and straightened it without the pain. Sitting in their midst for hours at a time, I heard grown women gossip about men and husbands and other women and jobs they hated and grown children who had turned out no good and a Temptations concert at the Howard Theatre. Going to the beauty parlor was as much about growing up and being initiated into the culture of grown Black women as it was about my hair. And everyone else's. The beauticians could brutally joke about women with short hair. That was the worst sin, for a woman's worth in the Black community, and all over the world, is determined by the length of her hair. "Good hair"—in case I didn't know by now—was straight, thick, and long. In the beauty parlor, I felt grown up and accepted into the real world of Black hair culture, with the caveat that I knew mine would never be good enough. All the women in my community who were considered the most beautiful had straight hair, women like Lena Horne and Dorothy Dandridge. Where would I fit in, how would I fit in, with my short, coarse hair and brown skin? And even when my hair was straightened, it always "went back" to its natural state. In a reprise of the famous test by sociologist Kenneth Clark that revealed that little Black girls chose White dolls over Black dolls, when little Black boys were tested to see which dolls they preferred, the boys routinely chose the Black dolls, which all had smooth hair, because, they said, of their hair. For boys, the magic of straight hair could triumph over the negative connotations of brown skin.

What all this tells us is that hair is not benign, it is important and potent. In the book *Hair Story: Untangling the Roots*

*of Black Hair in America*, Lori L. Tharps and Ayana D. Byrd
cite the work of the anthropologist Sylvia Ardyn Boone, who
found that among the Mende tribe of Sierra Leone, "'big
hair, plenty of hair, much hair,' were the qualities every
woman wanted," and that "unkempt, 'neglected,' or 'messy'
hair implied that a woman either had loose morals or was
insane." Traditionally in the Black community, mothers were
and still are judged by the state of their daughter's hair. I
remember as a child the worst judgments of adult women being reserved for women whose daughters left the house with
"nappy" or indifferently braided hair. This was a dereliction
of parental duty that was considered nearly a form of child
abuse. A *Washington Post* article about a White gay couple
who had adopted a little Black girl cited an incident in which
a Black woman, seeing the child on the subway with her two
dads, could no longer bear the sight of her amateurish braids
and left her seat and began braiding the girl's hair.

For Black women, hair is not just our crowning glory, it
is an expression of our souls. The furor over the hair of the
young Olympic gymnast Gabrielle Douglas in the summer
of 2012 was largely a Black female reaction to what some
women saw as her "nappy hair." The young teenager gave a
brilliant performance, and yes, at times, with the exertion
required, her hair did not look as "neat" as her White team-
mates'. Twitter and Facebook exploded with negative comments from some Black women, prompting a mainstream

media discussion about Black women and their hair. Media as diverse as the *Huffington Post*, the *Daily Beast*, and *Us Weekly* covered the controversy over what a small but vocal sect of the Black female online community dubbed "messy" and "unkempt" hair. Douglas's mother was forced to respond to the court of public opinion and post on the Internet explanations and apologies for "what happened to Gabby's hair."

Traditionally, among many African groups, a person's spirit is supposedly nestled in the hair, and the hairdresser is considered the most trustworthy individual in society. Clearly, African American attitudes about hair have been shaped by our living and vibrant cultural heritage, as well as by the requirements of trying to overcome oppressive attitudes about how Black people should look, think, act, and live. The "beauty parlor" and the barbershop remain among the most important institutions in the Black community. They are where we gossip, make friends, and talk politics outside the view and dominion of Whites, and where in many cases we have our confidence and self-esteem restored.

In the 1960s, hair became a form of political and cultural statement and protest. Everyone was letting his or her hair grow

> *Traditionally, among many African groups, a person's spirit is supposedly nestled in the hair, and the hairdresser is considered the most trustworthy individual in society.*

out or grow long, men and women, Black and White. The first time I ever liked my face or my hair was when I looked at myself in the mirror the day that I got my natural. I was an eighteen-year-old freshman who had entered American University five months after the assassination of Dr. Martin Luther King Jr. The world was one of riots and rage and questioning everything from why Blacks had so little power, to why we were in Vietnam, to why Blacks had to look like Whites to be considered beautiful. It was a world of new kinds of questions and answers. Black suddenly became beautiful. I looked around and liked what I saw on the heads and on the faces of my Black female friends and peers who wore Afros. The natural hairstyle showcased their faces, and they were faces that seemed to be proud and confident. That is what I wanted to be. It was as if I had never before really seen my face that day I looked in the mirror. My first natural was a delicate, short, close-cropped affair, and the hair that I had hated and been on a quest to change suddenly seemed so lovely, so perfect. My family was aghast. I withstood teasing, and threats from my father to cut me off financially, all because of my hair. But for the first time in my life, I accepted my hair and myself.

The natural hairstyle ultimately inspired a resurgence of African-inspired hairdos: twists, cornrows, and locks that had a long history among Black women. This simple hairdo laid down a challenge to the central tenet of Black hair and all it stood for—that it was bad and should be rejected. The natural required care but not torturous care. And for me, the fact that my hair became the backdrop for my face, rather than the other way around, was so satisfying. The impact of the natural lasted about a decade. Then straight hair came back with a vengeance, while I kept my own hair natural, except for one or two times when I used a relaxer just for a change. But the chemicals always damaged my hair. The natural revealed, in ways that more traditional styles did not, what I now had come to know was an attractive face. It fit my busy lifestyle, and I liked the way I looked and felt wearing a natural—free and comfortable in my skin.

Whatever Black women do to their hair is controversial. The straightening of Black hair was controversial when first introduced at the turn of the twentieth century. The technique was loudly criticized by the Black elite, even though many of them had straight hair that afforded them higher levels of acceptance by Whites than other Blacks received. When Blacks moved north during the Great Migration, women with braided hair or unstraightened hair were criticized as "country" and considered an embarrassment to their recently migrated yet suddenly urbanized cousins. Fast-forward half a century, and the Afro and natural were in some corners criticized as unkempt and uncivilized. Even today, many feel that natural hair is questionable as a legitimate hairstyle. The talk show host Wendy Williams criticized the actress Viola Davis so virulently for wearing her hair in a natural style to the Oscars in 2012, you would have thought she had attended the ceremony with a bag on her head. Recently, I was invited to speak to a group of high school girls who wanted to wear natural hair and who had formed a support group to sustain them in their decision. They shared heartbreaking stories of parents and friends who questioned their judgment because of this choice and predicted all manner of ruin and disaster for these girls. Yes, Black women have been fired from corporate jobs for wearing cornrows (too ethnic) and for putting a blond streak in their hair at Hooters (Black women don't have blond hair). But the CEO of Xerox, Ursula Burns, wears a natural, and the real world of corporations has learned to make room for constantly changing expressions of racial and ethnic beauty, even as there is ever-present pushback, attempting to enforce a unitary beauty and hair standard. This twixt and tween is simply called reality.

Black women never really win the hair wars. We keep getting hit by incoming fire from all sides. Today our hair is as much of a conundrum as ever. While Black women spend more on their hair than anyone else, they are routinely less satisfied with results. Weaves, wigs, and extensions are mainstream, from the heads of high school girls to those of TV reality series housewives.

The cultural skirmishes over the significance of Michelle

Obama's hair and her look signifies just how important these questions still are. Just as in the minds of many Whites, there is the image of the "angry" Black man and "angry" Black woman (usually brown to black in skin tone, hands on hips, often but not always full figured), there is also "angry" Black hair. During the 2008 presidential election campaign, when the *New Yorker* magazine wanted to capture the paranoia that some Whites felt about a possible Obama presidency, the magazine ran a cover that featured Barack Obama dressed as a Muslim cleric and Michelle Obama sporting an Afro, an AK-47 strapped over her shoulders, and a "shut your mouth" glare. While clearly the cover was meant to parody mindless racism, many across the political spectrum took offense.

*Black women never really win the hair wars. We keep getting hit by incoming fire from all sides.*

As First Lady, Michelle Obama has been crowned, quite justly, an American queen of style and glamour. She is considered by many ordinary folk, as well as those who are the arbiters of fashion and style, to be beautiful and elegant and a premier symbol of American female beauty, as influential as Jacqueline Kennedy. And her hair, whether it's bone straight that day, straight but curly, or straight and shiny, has been an endorsement of conventional, acceptable styles. Just as Barack Obama declared that he was president of "all America,"

Michelle Obama's hair has been accepted from sea to shining sea. All but the most hardcore Black cultural nationalists, who long to see a Black woman with an Afro in the White House, or White racists who have in Internet chat rooms called the First Lady and her daughters "gorillas," agree that the First Lady is the one Black woman in America who has won the hair wars. And beyond the question of hair, who would have imagined a beautiful brown-skinned, identifiably Black woman as the nation's First Lady? OK, the revolution just got televised.

Yet the controversy continues generation after generation. The cultural tumult is inspired, I feel, by the questions that continually haunt Black people. Questions that years of activism, protest, and progress have failed to answer in ways we can uniformly accept: Who are we? What makes us "authentic" Black people? What is *our* standard of beauty, and where are the roots of that beauty to be found? We can't agree on the answers, and we both accept and reject the conclusions forced on us by the larger White society. These questions spring from our position as both central to American culture and perennially marginalized by it.

And there are the other questions that hair leads to as well, about femininity, questions that haunt women of all shades, hues, and races. Why do we have to live under the tyranny of a global doctrine that posits femininity in the length and straightness of a woman's hair? Especially when real beauty, the kind that can light up a room literally and figuratively, radiates from within? Black women, like women all over the world, live imprisoned by a cultural belief system about beauty and hair whose time should have passed.

Today my natural is full of gray hairs, and I love it and my face more than ever, as the battle about Black hair rages on. I often wonder if, with my college degree, my status as a published author and educator who has worn natural hair for over forty years, I am too dismissive and critical of the reasons why so many Black women care so deeply about the state of their hair. I care about my hair too and have frankly chosen the natural as a form of adornment and statement.

But as I said, if you are a Black woman, hair is serious business. My hairphobic sisters have gotten the same message that I received relentlessly as a young girl: my natural hair is bad and it could exact a potentially high price if I choose to expose it and exult in it. I have just always been willing to pay the price. But my sisters know that with straight hair they are acceptable in the corporate world. They see high-profile celebrities like Beyoncé disguise her natural hair with a head full of synthetic hair and rule the world. They have lost jobs because they chose to wear braids. They know that many Black men prefer long, straight hair, and they don't care what Black women do to get it.

Yet I am deeply conflicted as I assess the young Black girl making minimum wage at McDonald's, sporting a weave that could easily cost thousands of dollars a year to maintain, money that, yes, I dare to say, she could use to go to college. Certainly a college degree would have a more positive long-term impact on her career goals than a weave. I am conflicted as well by the sight of a Black female professional wearing a wig whose locks reach the middle of her back. All of this is squishy, squirmy, and very difficult to write and speak out loud, for I am violating the racial rules about not airing dirty linen in public and the rule that says sisterhood trumps truths that may be hard to handle. I feel narrow minded and judgmental, when all I really want is a world where Black women are healthy and have healthy hair that does not put them in the poorhouse, cause health problems, or reinforce the idea that they have to look White to be valued. And this does not mean that I want a world of Black women who have hair that only looks like mine.

Yet who I am to judge? Who am I to assume that women who invest hundreds and sometimes thousands of dollars in synthetic hair don't or can't have as much racial pride as I do? Maybe they know something I don't, that what's on your head is not necessarily a barometer of what is in your mind. I know that Black women make these hair choices for reasons beyond reflexive conformity to White beauty standards, reasons such as convenience and the practical need to "fit in" to a prevailing White standard of beauty for the sake of their careers. I know that Black women are damned no matter what we do to our hair. And we are damned, ironically and most cruelly, by our own people, who are not often the ones who hire and fire, but are the ones who accept us into or push us out of the tribe. But I know too how deeply the wounds of racism and self-hatred have burrowed into the souls of Black men and women. I still hear too many Black women, and Black girls of all ages, talk obsessively among themselves, on the Internet, in social media, and face-to-face, about their desire for "good hair" and how much they fear having "bad hair." I am still waiting for that conversation to cease. I have been waiting all my life.

# Sister

. . . . . . . . . . . . . . . . . . . . . . . . . . . . . . . . . . . . . . . . . . . . . . . . . . . . .

## ANNE LAMOTT

On a trip to St. Louis a number of years ago, something for which I'd waited a lifetime happened: people asked me how they could get their hair to look like mine. I have dreadlocks now. I finally have fabulous hair. Now, you may need a little background on this to help you see why this means such a great deal to me: you've got to realize I grew up with men and boys asking me if I'd stuck my finger in a light socket. Of course, it's one thing when you're a twelve-year-old girl with nappy hair and the older boys ask if you've stuck your finger in the light socket; this is certainly exhilarating enough and could give a girl enough confidence literally to *soar* through puberty. But it's another when you have to keep fending off the question well into your twenties and thirties. Once at a funeral, an old friend of the woman who'd died actually asked me if I'd stuck my finger in a socket. At a funeral! And his wife had to stand beside him trying to look as if this were the most amusing thing you could possibly say at a funeral. I looked at her with compassion, and then at him rather blankly, and said as gently as I could, "What a rude, rude thing to say."

I was a towheaded child with bushy urchin hair. My father and some of my chosen mothers thought my hair was beautiful, but they were about the only ones who did. I got teased a lot. My mother took me to get it straightened for a while; I slept on rollers for years, brushed it into pigtails that I tied with pretty ribbons, set the bangs with enough gel to caulk a bathtub, and finally got it cut into an Afro in the late sixties. It looked better, but I loved having bangs, and they seemed to be forever a pipe dream.

Industrial-strength mousse came along in my twenties and I could moussify my hair and bangs into submission with this space-age antifrizz shit that may turn out someday to have been carcinogenic. I used to worry about this, but then I'd think, I don't really care as long as they don't take it off the market.

When I first started going to St. Andrew, most of the thirty or so women at my church who are African American processed their hair, and still do. A few wear short Afros, a few wear braided extensions; but mostly they get it straightened or flattened against their heads into marcel waves. When I got dreadlocks a few years ago, the other women were ambivalent at first. I think it made them a little afraid for me.

Dreadlocks make people wonder if you're trying to be rebellious. It's not as garbling and stapled as a tongue stud, say, or as snaky as tattoos. But dreadlocks make you look a little like Medusa, because they writhe and appear to have a life of their own, and that's scary. These women at my church love me more than life itself, and they want me to move safely through the world. They want me to pass. So they worried, and slipped the name of black beauty salons into our conversations.

When I first started coming to this church, I wore my hair like I'd worn it for years, shoulder length and ringletty—or at any rate, ringletty if there was an absence of wind, rain, or humidity. In the absence of weather, with a lot of mousse on hand, I could get it to fall just right so that it would not be too frizzy and upsetting—although "fall" is perhaps not the right word. "Appear to fall" is close. "Shellacked into the illusion of 'falling'" is even closer. Weather is the enemy. I could leave the house with bangs down to my eyebrows, moussed and frozen into place like the plastic sushi in the windows of Japanese restaurants,

> *Dreadlocks make people wonder if you're trying to be rebellious. It's not as garbling and stapled as a tongue stud, say, or as snaky as tattoos.*

and after five minutes in rain or humidity, I'd look like Ronald McDonald.

Can you imagine the hopelessness of trying to live a spiritual life when you're secretly looking up at the skies not for illumination or direction but to gauge, miserably, the odds of rain? Can you imagine how discouraging it was for me to live in fear of weather, of drizzle or downpour? Because Christianity is *about* water: "Everyone that thirsteth, come ye to the waters." It's about baptism, for God's sake. It's about full immersion, about falling into something elemental and *wet*. Most of what we do in worldly life is geared toward our staying dry, looking good, not going under. But in baptism, in lakes and rain and tanks and fonts, you agree to do something that's a little sloppy because at the same time it's also holy, and absurd. It's about surrender, giving in to all those things we can't control; it's a willingness to let go of balance and decorum and get *drenched*.

There's something so tender about this to me, about being willing to have your makeup wash off, your eyes tear up, your nose start to run. It's tender partly because it harkens back to infancy, to your mother washing your face with love and lots of water, tending to you, making you clean all over again. And in the Christian experience of baptism, the hope is that when you go under and you come out, maybe a little disoriented, you haven't dragged the old day along behind you. The hope, the belief, is that a new day is upon you now.

A day when you are emboldened to take God at God's word about cleanness and protection: "When thou passeth through the water, I will be with thee; and through the rivers, they shall not overflow thee."

Obviously, when you really want this companionship and confidence but you're worried about your bangs shrinking up like fern fronds, you've got a problem on your hands.

Furthermore, I don't think you're supposed to devote so much of your prayer life to the desperate hope that there not be any weather. Also, to the hope that no one trick you into getting into a convertible and then suddenly insist on putting the top down. Because I tell you, you take a person with fluffy wiry hair like mine and you put her in a convertible with the top down, the person gets out of the car looking like Buckwheat. Or Don King. It helps in one way to wear a hat, but when you take it off you have terrible hat hair—it looks like a cartoon mouse has been driving a little steamroller around your head. And you can't wear a scarf or you end up looking like your Aunt Bev. So you have to pick—Don King, or Bev.

So that's the background. Now I have dreadlocks, long blondish dreadlocks, and some of the people of St. Louis were asking me how they could get their hair to dread. All right, not many of them, but two of them, two straight white normal-looking middle-aged people. Mostly, people see someone with dreadlocks, especially a white person with dreadlocks, and assume that the person's hair carries with it a position or a message—the message being, Maybe you don't have as many prejudices against me as you do against black people, but you should. Most people, if asked, might wonder if perhaps dreadlocks are somewhat unpatriotic—isn't it unpatriotic not to comb your hair? The tangles are so funky, and who knows, they may harbor bugs and disease. Perhaps to some people dreadlocks indicate confusion of thought and character: good children have shiny combed hair, while bad children, poor children, loser kids, have bushy hair.

*Most people, if asked, might wonder if perhaps dreadlocks are somewhat unpatriotic—isn't it unpatriotic not to comb your hair?*

But two people in St. Louis stopped me on the street and asked for instructions on how to get their hair to look like mine.

Eight years after I joined St. Andrew, I moved to a new neighborhood north of where we'd been living. The bad news was that there was more weather there. Hotter weather, more humid weather, fern-frond bangs weather. The good news was that a large, beautiful radical African American Buddhist professor named Marlene Jones Schoonover lived there too, and she had the most beautiful dreadlocks—lovely playful dreadlocks, carefully groomed, like wild plants in well-tended rows.

Soon after moving there, I became the Democratic precinct leader for our neighborhood, and I used to pass her house as I made my rounds. She not only had hair I loved but a glorious bright overgrown garden like one you'd find on the grounds of Clown College. One time I stopped to talk to her when she was out in her yard picking flowers, and I admired her dreads out loud. "You ought to do it," she said. "My daughter and I did it as an act of civil rights. And we could help you do it too."

I said that sounded just great—but I knew I wasn't going to follow up. First of all, I felt it was presumptuous to appropriate a black style for my own liberation. But mostly when I thought about having dreadlocks, I felt afraid and disloyal. Dreadlocks would be a way of saying I was no longer going to play with the rules of mainstream white beauty. It meant that I was no longer going to even try and blend. It was a way of saying that I know what kind of hair I have, I know what it looks like, and I am going to stop trying to pretend it's different than that. That I was going to celebrate instead.

But I was not ready; I continued to moussify.

No one knew the effort it took to make my hair look like it hadn't taken any effort at all.

I'd pass Marlene in her garden, and she'd look up from her work and say, "You have such beautiful hair."

"Oh, thank you," I'd say, and paw the ground.

One day she said, "I *love* your hair." And then she went on, "Picture Jesus with hair just like yours." But I couldn't, any more than I could imagine him with braces on his teeth or short hairy legs. That's how deeply I had come to believe that my hair was ugly.

On the other hand, I *could* immediately see Jesus with dreadlocks flowing down his back. And I saw that it would be an act of both triumph and surrender to give up trying to have straighter hair. And that surrender means you get to come on over to the winning side.

But I *still* wasn't ready to do it.

Then two things happened. One was that all of a sudden I couldn't stop thinking of something Pammy said right before she died, when she was in a wheelchair, wearing a wig to cover her baldness. We were at Macy's. I was modeling a short dress for her that I thought my boyfriend would like. But then I asked whether it made me look big in the hips, and Pammy said, as clear and kind as a woman can be, "Annie? You really don't have that kind of time." And—slide trombone, bells, rim shot—I *got* it, deep in my being. While walking by Marlene's garden, Pammy's words suddenly rang through the chambers of my mind.

So I kept thinking, How much longer am I going to think about my hair more often than about things in the world that matter? I kept passing Marlene's house. She'd be out watering her crazy clown garden. We'd talk about politics, our children, and God. Then we'd talk about hair. "Call me," she'd say, "when you're ready." She knew how scared I was.

One day I said, "I think I'm getting there."

"Princess be about to *arrive*," she said.

The second thing was that right around that time, I saw *The Shawshank Redemption*, where at the end, the character played by Tim Robbins escapes from prison via the sewers after serving time for a crime he didn't commit. He emerges from the pipes of the prison into a rushing rain-swollen river and he staggers through the current with his face turned toward the sky, his arms held up to heaven as the rains pour down.

I sat in the movie theater and cried for a while. Then I started to smile, because it occurred to me that if I were the prisoner being baptized by the torrential rain, half my mind would be on how much my bangs were going to shrink up after they dried.

I went home that night and I called Marlene. "OK, baby," I said. "I'm ready."

The next day she and her dreadlocked teenage daughter came over to my house with a little jar of beeswax, which would hold the baby dreads in place until they could start tangling themselves together into strands. Marlene sat me down in the kitchen. She and her daughter sectioned off my hair, twisted it into long strands that almost looked braided, and glued it in place with the wax. It took a couple of hours, and I was scared almost the whole time. We listened to gospel and reggae for inspiration. I cried a little—I had never let people enter into my hair weirdness with me, had never let anyone help me before, had never believed I could get free. I let them work on me, and after a while I thought of the sacredness of animals grooming each other. I felt the connection and the tenderness, the reciprocal healing offered by the laying on of hands. The two women twisted, daubed, smoothed my hair, practical and gentle at the same time; there aren't many opportunities for this left, away from the sickbed. Marlene worked with the grave sense that we were doing something meaningful—politically, spiritually, aesthetically. And her quiet daughter worked with bouncy joyful efficiency, bopping along to the reggae beat. When they were done, I looked beautiful—royal, shy, groomed. Beautiful. Strange. Mulatto.

Who will love me now? I wondered. Will anyone want to stroke my hair again? I didn't know the answer, so this act was like taking a vow of chastity. And I didn't care. I just wanted to stroke my hair myself.

The dreads are so cool; no wonder two people in St. Louis wanted my secret. Like snowflakes, each dreadlock is different, has its own configuration, its own breadth and feel. It's like having very safe multiple personalities. It's been twenty years since that day Marlene and her daughter first twisted them into vines, and they have grown way past my shoulders down my back. Sometimes I wear them up, sometimes down. I used to look at people with normal white people's hair, and their bangs always stayed long and they got to hide behind that satin curtain, and I was jealous. But now my bangs are always long too. I peered out at St. Louis from behind my dreadlocks, as through a beautiful handmade fence, in the drizzle, in the wind, in the rain.

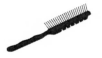

# Frizzball

PATRICIA VOLK

I have thousands of enemies. That's not in my head. It's *on* my head. I'm talking follicles. The average person has 130,000. Follicles can be friendly or you can spend your entire life as I have, duking it out with them every single humidiphobic day.

This was not always the case. I was born with "naturally curly hair." It did everything my mother wanted it to. People stopped her on the street. "Naturally curly!" they'd gasp. "She's *blessed*!" Pity my poor straight-haired sister. Jo Ann was pressed into biannual perms. Every six months she'd pass a chemical-scented afternoon at Best and Company, wired to black rods dangling from a chrome dome that shot electricity through her hair. She'd come home with a ridged coif that blasted out at the sides like Clarabell's. It took two weeks to calm down. After a month, it verged on normal, almost as if she too were blessed with naturally curly hair.

Something happened. One day in summer camp, bored during rest hour, I took the manicuring scissors out of my sewing kit and, without a mirror, gave myself a haircut. It was work. Manicuring scissors can't handle much more than a cuticle. But I had an hour and I kept at it, watching wispy letter *C*s waft down on my Camp Red Wing blanket.

"WHAT HAVE YOU DONE?" Mom shrieked on visiting day.

She marks the change in my hair to that self-inflicted haircut. It was no longer naturally curly. It grew back pure frizz. This dovetailed with the onset of puberty. Much as it alters your hips and breasts, puberty can reconfigure your follicles too. So can chemotherapy. Friends who have endured it invariably like their new hair better. Straights became curly. Curlies became straight. That said, I don't recommend chemotherapy as a hair treatment, although it's the only one I haven't tried.

From the ages of twelve through twenty-one, I slept in rollers with Scotch tape across my bangs. I left for college with my very own salon hood dryer. I spent my honeymoon in Barbados without getting my hair wet once. I've had my hair wound tight around my head like a turban at the late Louis-Guy D' on East Fifty-Seventh Street. Kenneth yanked it taut on rollers the width of a French bread. Philip torched it at Crimpers, once searing my temple so badly it left a scar the size of a calcium pill. Ralph at Bumble and Bumble stretched and fried it. I endured potash and lye and human Mexican placenta in a roach-ridden emporium above a strip joint on Broadway. Irons and flat wands. Cornrows with beads, cornrows without. Diet control. Dryers that parched my eyeballs. Sleeping with a stocking stretched over my head. Do-rags. Dippity-do and Dixie Peach. Beer and Miss Jessie's. Gels and sprays. Alberto VO5 and Toni home perms in reverse. I draw the line at the Japanese treatment. Formaldehyde is not for the living. Once, channeling the very beautiful Bernadette Peters, I visited a salon that specializes in curls. There are two in New York: Ouidad and Devachan. Both use a similar technique: drenching a wet head with their product, followed by scrunching (never combing or brushing), then letting the hair air-dry, which takes forever. You're not just waiting for water to evaporate. You've got four ounces of goop in there too. In theory, this results in the much-coveted "curl differentiation." The curls separate. You have countless Shirley Temple springs. It's a look. It just isn't mine. And you have to do it every day or it gets mashed.

Three years ago, I tried the keratin treatment. How strange it is to get exactly what you want, exactly what you hoped for. Keratin works. My hair was straight in a way it had never been. Stick straight and shiny. It was life-changing. I immediately stopped having good days and bad days based on my hair. For as long as the keratin lasted (three months), I woke up flawless.

I pulled my hair back in a scrunchy and it stayed there. I swam! I played tennis! I washed my hair and was good to go! A whole new world opened up, a world without hair anxiety. Men gazed at me with longing on the street. Maître d's led me to the best table. Doormen scurried to take my shopping bags. Smiling sales assistants elbowed each other to wait on me. The straight world was a new and better place. How different from my curly life, where people assume if my hair is out of control I am too. Once a stranger came up to me at a party, patted my mop, and said, "Tell me. I've got to know. Do you have straight pubic hair?"

Fact: not a single member of my family has curly hair. My mother gave up smoking during her pregnancy, and I blame my frizz on that jolt to her system. How I longed for her sleek Grace Kelly smoothness! It skipped a generation. Thank God my daughter has my mother's hair, not mine. I call it "metronome hair." It sways in time with her hips when she walks. I doubt Polly ever rolls out of bed, faces the bathroom mirror, and says, What fresh hell is this?

HIGH-FUNCTIONING HAIR OBSESSIVES rarely go it alone. We have a team. The products, the people. Right this very minute, under my sink, for when I go curly: John Frieda Frizz Ease Clearly Defined gel ($6), John Frieda Frizz Ease Dream Curls conditioner ($11), John Frieda Frizz Ease moisture barrier firm hold hairspray ($11), John Frieda Frizz

Ease Unwind Curls calming cream ($6), Moroccanoil curl-defining cream ($36), Moroccanoil intense curl cream ($45), Kevin.Murphy Anti.Gravity oil-free volumizer ($37), Coppola color care shampoo ($15), Coppola color care conditioner ($20), Living Proof No Frizz restyling spray ($16).

*High-functioning hair obsessives rarely go it alone. We have a team. The products, the people.*

For summertime, when I spring for the keratin treatment: Louis Licari Ionic Color Preservation System styling foam gel ($24), Louis Licari volumizing daily root lift for fine hair ($14), Lasio Hypersilk smoothing balm ($34), Living Proof Amp$^2$ instant texture volumizer ($26), Living Proof styling cream ($29), Oribe dry texturizing spray ($42), and Rene Furterer Karité repairing serum ($30). I am one minuscule reason why the hair care industry, according to Goldman Sachs, is worth $38 billion a year in products alone. (Skin care comes in at $24 billion, and makeup, a mere $18 billion.)

In addition to products, I have a human team: I go to Louis Licari in New York every month for color with Kazu. Louis Licari, formerly a painter, is famous primarily for color, NBC's "Ambush Makeover," and the latest hair tech. His salon isn't a "scene," even though movie stars are getting washed in the sink next to mine. The people are authentic and friendly. I get cut by Bridgette or Max or Devi or Igor. Then they blow my hair out. And in the summer, a.k.a. Frizzball Season, Arsen gives me the Coppola keratin treatment, leaving my hair Joan Baez straight, ever the goal. I only do it once a year because it costs $500, and the older I get, the more the hair of my dreams ages me. So I have to choose: Do I want to look like Margaret Atwood, frizzy and old? Or Georgia O'Keeffe, straight and old? Briefly, in the hippie-dippie seventies, my hair was hot. Think of Julie Christie in *McCabe and Mrs. Miller*. But controlled hair and only controlled hair is in now. If you check beautyblitz.com, the "One Click From Gorgeous" website for everything beauty, you will notice that if a Beauty Blitz nape bun is messy, it is by design. If a tendril flops, it flops with precision. There is no room for frizzball on beautyblitz.com.

It's happy-making to find a Library of America newsletter in the mail. What a great organization. The LOA reprints the work of the best American authors in handsome acid-free editions. Supporters attend book events where many of them are photographed. Reading the latest issue, I realized something strange. Of the eighty-eight women pictured, only one had remotely curly hair. That would be the timeless beauty Jeannette Watson Sanger. Her hair had waves and bounce. No one had frizz.

According to *Scientific American*, there is no difference between hair and fur. So why do *Homo sapiens* come with such variety? In the animal kingdom, you don't see frizzy horses or kinky monkeys. You don't see straight-haired poodles or lanky-haired sheep. Was our species given bigger brains so we could worry about our hair? Hello, Darwin? Why us? Why me?

Sometimes I think of asking Kazu to bleach my hair Marilyn blond, then convincing Igor to cut it short enough to spike like Laurie Anderson's. I'd use enough glop to keep the spikes impervious and never think about my hair again. But I'm a coward. That said, please do not feel sorry for me. I've almost learned to live with it. And if I didn't fret about my hair, something else would take its place. I believe we are born with a cup of

*Was our species given bigger brains so we could worry about our hair? Hello, Darwin? Why us? Why me?*

affliction and it is our destiny to keep that cup filled at all times. If something terrible happens, I forget about my hair. When my parents got sick, my hair was a nonissue. But here I am, an orphan now, back to worrying about my hair. Not that frizzy doesn't have an upside. On an airplane, I never have to ask for a pillow. In winter, my hair traps so much body heat I rarely need a hat. Caught in the rain, I look *better* as my hair flattens. Best of all, my toddler grandsons love it. They squeal and pat it and lose their hands in it. If there's anything better than Jack, Sam, and Miles patting my hair and laughing, tell me. You can't, can you.

# And Be Sure to Tell Your Mother

ALEX KUCZYNSKI

**M**y tribe is a hairless one. Two years ago, when I spit into a plastic vial and sent my saliva to 23andMe to have my genetic history mapped, one of the traits that came back—apart from being, oddly, closely related to Dr. Oz—was the following: "You are from people with the least amount of body hair on earth." There was a map and an arrow pointing to a dot, somewhere between northern Europe and Scandinavia, and it basically said: You are here, and hairless. So when I grew pubic hair—probably sometime around eighteen years old—it was not a big deal. I never thought of grooming or plucking or shaving or bleaching; it seemed unnecessary and there wasn't very much to work with anyway. I also didn't own a bikini or have sex until my twenties—I know: *Freak!*—so there was no point.

When I was twenty-four, this changed. I found myself in Istanbul, in a hammam, at the suggestion of my friend Verkin. In the domed steam room, the attendants scrubbed me raw, massaged me, flayed me with scented tree branches, and anointed me. Then the *tellak*—the one who scrubs and flays and greases you up—took me by the hand to a private room off to the side and started asking pleasant questions in Turkish. She seemed encouraging, so I nodded affirmatively, even though the only phrases I understood in Turkish at the time were "cherry juice," "Where is the toilet?" and "Enough with the rugs already."

With an athletic abruptness, she flipped my legs over my head and started applying some sort of honeyed mixture to the hair of my pubic region. Within minutes, helpless to stop but cautiously willing, I was bare as a baby. Verkin wandered in to check on me. I lay on the marble slab, supine, stunned, stripped, feeling like a simultaneously pornographic and infantilized female version of the Lamentation of Christ.

"*Çok güzel,*" Verkin said in Turkish to the attendant, who smiled brightly at the praise of her work. *Very beautiful.* I will never forget those words. I associate them with shock and vulnerability—and chafing. I arrived back in the hotel, and my boyfriend remarked that I looked like an enormous eight-year-old, and we continued on our journey, which had started in the ecstatic hedonism of the Greek islands, through Turkey and on into the bound and covered-up monasticism of Syria, where I wore long sleeves, a long skirt, and a head scarf that covered my face. Underneath, my skin was naked, no hair below my eyebrows longer than a grain of rice. I would learn that in Islam, pubic and underarm hair is considered unclean for both sexes and is routinely shaved or waxed. In Syria, even though I felt like a filthy sex goddess/giant eight-year-old, I actually fit right in.

Years later, I often reflect on the paradox of the American woman, influenced by porn-star culture, stripping off her pubic hair, coerced into a state of enforced genital infancy, and her similarity to Muslim women all over the world. They spend their entire adult lives never seeing a pubic hair on their bodies— but in their case, it is for religious reasons. In one culture, porn rules; in the other, God. The result is the same.

In the past two decades, with the absorption of pornography into the American mainstream—pole-dancing aerobics classes, Abercrombie thong underwear for the six- to eight-year-old set, suburban couples making homemade porn movies, nip slips on television, Miley Cyrus basically doing anything—pubic hair has become a quasi-public marker of the self, a talisman of one's essential style, even though presumably very few people see what your pubic hair actually looks like. Books have been written about the many possibilities for pubic coifs. Women celebrities talk about their pubic hair in an open and casual way, and I am still not used to hearing it. It always strikes me as misguided, as if they believe this open kind of conversation is an empowering feminist move, wresting sexual discussion away from men and using it as their own device to convey sexual bravura. I found it profoundly embarrassing when Jennifer Love Hewitt revealed to the talk show host George Lopez that she had "vajazzled" her vulva. "A friend of mine Swarovski-crystalled my precious lady—and it shined like a disco ball," she said, adding, "Women should vajazzle their vajayjays." It made her feel better, she said, after a nasty breakup.

*Women celebrities talk about their pubic hair in an open and casual way, and I am still not used to hearing it.*

A brief aside on what vajazzling entails: someone strips all the hair off your vulva, labia, and anus and then glues crystals or pearls in some sort of decorative motif in place of the hair. (*Vajazzling* is a play on the words *vagina* and *Bedazzler*, which is a home appliance used to fasten rhinestones, studs, and patches to clothes and other material.) First of all: Don't google this. (Or the phrase "Willie Nelson vagina tattoo.") You can't unsee it. (And you really can't unsee that Willie Nelson tattoo. It haunts me.) Second: Why would you want to put glue all over your vulva? How can you function while coated, privately, in rhinestones? Exercise? Make love? The actress was, of course, promoting a book about "female empowerment." What I saw was a desperate celebrity trying to make headlines before she U-boated out of sight forever.

I WAS MORTIFIED when I heard Gwyneth Paltrow publicly ramble on about growing a "seventies bush." Why do I want to know this? Does she think it makes her seem more human, more natural, more down to earth, to talk about her wild and woolly pubic hair? In fact, it seems overly thought out, processed through the neural pathways of seventeen public relations executives, and delivered on a talk show for the sole purpose of having people (just like I am doing now! Brava!) repeat it.

In my twenties and thirties, I worked as a reporter and often subjected myself to projects that involved the body. There was a graphic front-page story for the *New York Observer* about my experience with colonic irrigation. I wrote a piece for the *New York Times* about women experimenting with Viagra for enhanced sexual gratification (I believe I was the first *New York Times* reporter to get the word *horny* into the paper of record). Later, I was asked by a women's magazine to get a "vajacial" and write about the experience. During the treatment, an aesthetician performed a cleansing "facial" treatment on my vulva, explaining why it was necessary: so many women get ingrown hairs from waxing, or they have irritated skin from dying their pubic hair hot pink or blue (often using a product called Betty Beauty, for "the hair down there"), or the glue from vajazzling creates clogged pores. The most disturbing part of the "vajacial" was that, unlike during a facial, when one's mouth is presumably closed to receive relaxing treatment of the entire facial region, one's mouth is not closed during a vajacial, and so you might find yourself making uncomfortable conversation with the vajacialist while she is nicking at ingrown hairs, pointing out areas that might benefit from a special vulva rejuvenation serum or from Pink Daisy labia bleaching cream, or suggesting the most gentle organic anal bleach (Dr. Pinks anal bleaching cream)—for next time.

TRIMMING OR REMOVING pubic hair—the term for the preference for hairless genitals is *acomoclitism*—has long been a custom in many cultures for medical, religious, or cultural reasons. In ancient Egypt, removing hair meant fewer lice infestations. Greeks and Romans commonly removed all their body hair for aesthetic reasons. In Muslim cultures, depilation (removing the hair above the skin) or epilation (removing the entire hair including the root below the skin) is a basic hygienic ritual, on par with toothbrushing.

*The art and practice of pubic-hair maintenance traveled with Islam through northern Africa to Europe.*

In the sixteenth century, Michelangelo felt it was appropriate to create a David with stylized pubic hair, and by the eighteenth century, female pubic hair was often the centerpiece of Japanese erotic art, but it was typically not until the twentieth century that the Western tradition showed women with pubic hair. The celebrated nineteenth-century art critic John Ruskin, who seemed to have learned all he knew about women from art, not life, was so put off by his new wife's body on their honeymoon—some think it was the sight of her pubic hair—that the marriage was annulled, unconsummated, years later. Ruskin never did get used to the notion of pubic hair and may have died a virgin.

When Gustave Flaubert traveled to Egypt in the 1840s, he marveled at the women's acomoclitic state: "The shaved cunts make a strange effect," he wrote in his notes. "The flesh is as hard as bronze." After an encounter with a prostitute brokered by a friend, he offers the following: "Firm flesh, bronze arse, shaven cunt, dry though fatty; the whole thing gave the effect of a plague victim or a leperhouse."

The art and practice of pubic-hair maintenance traveled with Islam through northern Africa to Europe. In the 1860s, a Turkish diplomat commissioned Gustave Courbet to paint *L'Origine du monde*, with the proviso that the model brandish a full nest of pubic hair. The painting created a public scandal for its extremely naturalistic portrayal of a woman's bushy pubic mound and passed quietly through private collections before arriving at the Musée d'Orsay. It reminds me of the paintings of Lucian Freud and of the illustrations in *The Joy of Sex*, which struck my preadolescent friends and me as scandalous. Why? Not because of the dozens of exotic sexual arrangements before us, but because the bodies in the drawings of men and women thus engaged were *so* strangely hairy.

By the twentieth century, after clashing with Victorian prudishness, pubic-hair styling became—if not de rigueur—fully acceptable among the soigné Continental set. In 1930s Europe, the car dealer Baron Martin Stillman von Brabus reportedly shaved the pubic hair of his lover, Margaret, Duchess of Argyll, into a representation of the Mercedes-Benz logo.

That seems commonplace next to the choices we have today. One can get temporary tattoos on one's vulva, a practice called "vatooing." (And again, a gentle reminder: do not google the phrase "Willie Nelson vagina tattoo.") There is Betty Beauty dye, available in a rainbow of colors. Of course, the insidious vajazzling. Using hot wax and a detail trimmer (basically a tiny razor)—and if you so choose, a product such as Coochy shave cream—one can strip and shape one's hair into a variety of shapes, which have each earned nicknames in the common parlance of the trade. There is the vafro, the sphynx (also known as the Yul Brynner or full monty), the Bermuda Triangle, the football or the furry hoop, the flame (also known as the teardrop or princess), the diamond, the marquise, the landing strip, pencil line, and the minimalist. There is the Chaplin, the postage stamp, the Hitler, and the rattail. I recently spent a week on a nude beach in Maui and was less fascinated by the exquisite bodies than by the precision craft on display in everyone's pubic region, both women and men. The young women sported dynamic shapes and flamboyant dye jobs; the young men had waxed their bodies entirely and all their pubic hair, leaving just a strip over the top of their penises. The effect was to make their penises seem, well, huge, like long, dangling hoses. I know several men, heterosexual, who go in for full wax jobs of the areas that are most hairy, also known in the trade as "back, sack, and crack."

An entire current of contemporary art, pop culture, and commerce is dedicated to pubic hair. American Apparel recently featured storefront mannequins with fully hairy pubic regions. The artist Rhiannon Schneiderman created a series of portraits of herself wearing giant wigs over her pubic region. In England, Project Bush gathered together ninety-three women and photographed their pubic areas, in part to show young women and girls that it is entirely OK to have pubic hair. (One of Project Bush's creators was horrified to discover that girls as young as eleven and twelve were getting Brazilian bikini waxes.) The performance artist Julie Atlas Muz uses her vulva and vagina as a character in her work, Mr. Pussy. Mr.

*By the twentieth century, after clashing with Victorian prudishness, pubic-hair styling became— if not de rigueur— fully acceptable among the soigné Continental set.*

Pussy is made to speak, smoke cigarettes, and offer cultural commentary during "his" performances. Muz performs as Mr. Pussy to draw attention to the fact that the public sees feminine pubic hair as something frightening, something to be removed and waxed away. And in so doing, Muz recapitulates in her own way Denis Diderot's marvelous erotic novel *The Indiscreet Jewels*, in which a magic ring placed on a woman's finger will allow her vulva to speak, delivering her opinion and point of view "from the most honest part."

The trend that most disturbs me is women who have all their pubic hair lasered off, permanently, leaving them in a state of immortal prepubescence. I asked a group of such women why they would do such a thing—which is entirely irreversible—and the explanations made no sense to me. One woman said she did it because she was having her bikini line—just the sides—lasered off and why not just do the whole thing, for the slightest bit of price difference? Another said she never wanted to confront having gray pubic hair. Her comment reminded me of a friend who is going through horrible, excoriating chemotherapy, and who can't stand it when her fellow patients complain that the chemo treatments make them look so old. "I don't care about looking old," she says. "I just want the privilege of being able to *be old.*"

I've ventured into the weird world of pubic grooming a few times. After the Turkish hammam experience, it took my hair a full year to grow back. In my early thirties, my then four-year-old stepdaughter came to live with my husband and me for the first of many summers. I knew we would be changing into bathing suits together, and I knew her mother had voiced some doubt about whether the hair on my head—in the preferred vernacular, "the drapes"—was naturally that shade of shocking, unnatural blond. The truth is that it wasn't; the color had been foisted upon me at great expense by a Madison Avenue hairdresser. Before my stepdaughter's arrival, I decided to have a little fun with the situation. I turned on the TV, put my legs in the air and slathered Jolen cream bleach all over "the carpet." After two hours, all the hair on my body, from head to toe, correlated. It was all a matching, hideous shade of something my mother calls "pee-pee yellow."

A few days later, my four-year-old charge and I were changing in the beach cabana. She noticed that my pubic hair was a blinding Marilyn Monroe blond.

"Why is your hair there that color?" she said. "Wow."

"Well, of course, it's my natural hair color," I said, sliding into my bikini bottoms. Then I added: "And be sure to tell your mother."

Like many New York women, I've ventured into J Sisters, that torture palace of Brazilian hair waxing on Fifty-Seventh Street. And every time I have gone, I have stared up at the ceiling—at first glance it appears to be pressed metal, but the curling edges in the corner belie the fact that it is actually wallpaper, a shifty decorating ruse—and lay sweating and screaming as one of the sisters (or cousins, or friends, all of whose names begin with the letter *J*) strips the hair from an area on the body where pain seems sinisterly acute, and I have sworn every time: never again.

Finally, last year, after a run-in with an ingrown hair that resulted in an infection that required antibiotic treatment—I looked at my doctor in wonderment as he wrote out the prescription, and he said, shaking his head in a kind of rueful sorrow at the state of womanhood, "I have to do this about once a month"—I decided: no more. I like my hair. It keeps me warm in winter, prevents chafing during sports, and stores pheromonal scents. It provides padding. It marks me as a woman, not a child. I will not laser it away. I will keep it. And when it does turn gray, and later I hope white, maybe then I will dye it hot pink.

# Kozmic Hippie Hair Breakdown Blues

ROSIE SCHAAP

There she is on the cover of *Skeletons from the Closet*, the Grateful Dead's 1974 best-of record: Botticelli's Venus—clutching a red rose—wedged behind a skeleton. Painting nearly five hundred years before the Dead played its first show at Magoo's Pizza Parlor in 1965, in Menlo Park, California, Sandro Botticelli couldn't have anticipated that his Venus—that demure, pale-skinned paragon of Western femininity, with her mild gaze, her coy quasi smile, her head subtly, alluringly atilt—would become a model for the late twentieth-century second-wave hippie-girl ideal. And then, there's her hair: great waves of marigold and sunflower, long enough to conceal her sex, flowing, magnificent. How I once longed for hair like hers; how deeply and unhappily I knew I would never have it.

As a prototype of the perfect nature girl, Botticelli's Venus was one of the reasons I felt I never really cut it as a hippie chick, but she was not alone. My hair is naturally brown, and though about as curly as Botticelli's goddess's, it is inclined to frizz, in accordance with the practice of the hair of Jewish girls going back—in my imaginings anyway—to Sarah and Rebecca, Leah and Rachel. I suspect neither Joni Mitchell nor Michelle Phillips descend from that line, and if a girl following the Grateful Dead on tour couldn't have Venus hair, the next best thing was hair like theirs: blond and stick straight and parted in the middle, long and sleek and perfectly in place. My hair can only stand to grow so much, and then, when it has no more will, it stops. My frizz will rebel against even the most assiduous ministrations of the blow-dryer.

*How I once longed for hair like hers; how deeply and unhappily I knew I would never have it.*

With these real and mythical women as my impossible ideals, at age fifteen, in 1986, I flung myself—my whole, ardent, earnest young self—into the American counterculture of a generation prior. When I wasn't listening to the Dead, I was listening to folk music and psychedelia and boozy electric blues, to Bob Dylan and the Jim Kweskin Jug Band, to Jefferson Airplane and Jimi Hendrix and Janis Joplin and Crosby, Stills, and Nash (and sometimes Young). Other girls at my school prized their immaculate Benetton jerseys and stonewashed Guess jeans; I spent hours in thrift stores and little Indian dress shops in Greenwich Village, poring over racks of colorful garments, and wore layer upon layer of thin, block-printed cotton skirts, paired with tie-dyed T-shirts or embroidered Guatemalan tunics in temperate weather, or earthy, itchy, chunky Andean sweaters in the winter. I forswore shoes whenever possible (occasional concessions were made to a pair of tattered huaraches or Birkenstock sandals), the better to see the silver rings on my toes and the jangly little bells tied around my ankles, the better to feel the grass or sand or even pavement beneath my callused feet. Of course, I wore no makeup, and shaving was for suckers. I skipped school frequently to take part in Greenpeace and antiapartheid demonstrations or to retreat with friends to the Connecticut woods to drop acid. I doubt I thought too hard about it back then, but I still understood why I was doing what I was doing, beyond infuriating my mother: I felt out of place and out of time in Reagan's America, and the sixties seemed a better fit for me, even if my vision of the decade was romanticized and simpleminded and tenuous.

My efforts paid off: I dressed and acted the part so well that adults who'd actually lived through the era sometimes said that looking at me gave them flashbacks. Only my hair failed me. I could get the clothes right, the music right, the politics right, the lingo right, the vegetarian burritos right, even the twirling, spinning, kooky dancing right, but my hair always threatened to betray me as a sham hippie. I brushed it nightly in arduous, hour-long sessions in my incense-befogged and -scented bedroom, as though the more I brushed, the longer it would grow; as though there existed a hidden store of luxurious hair just under my scalp, and by brushing with real conviction I could summon it forth; as though some dormant, hidden hair was coiled in there like a snake to be charmed out of the clay urn of my head. I loved how when my hair was wet it seemed to settle and stretch, and how, if I angled my head back just so, I could feel it flick the middle of my back; this supplied an electric, tremendously pleasurable tingle. But when I straightened my neck again, it just barely grazed my shoulders, and the spell broke.

Those rare and tender moments when my hair made me feel like Joni Mitchell—or, more to the point, like certain graceful and desirable girls I knew in my Grateful Dead tour circle, the ones all the hippie boys circled like curious, feral dogs—were fleeting. Even in the world of Deadheads, which I had counted on to be more just and less orthodox where expectations of appearance based on gender were concerned, long (and preferably blond) hair equaled feminine beauty. In Janis Joplin, I identified a more realistic, if perhaps more dangerous, sixties icon upon whom to model myself. Her wild, reckless frizz was much more like my own hair; her brash, bawdy, hard-drinking, hard-living *Pearl* persona was easier for me to emulate than Joni's quieter, ladylike intensity.

Back then, we didn't know from karaoke, but a late-night session of lip-synching to a favorite song, played on a vinyl record, was a regular feature of high school parties in basement rec rooms. My big number was Joplin's "Piece of My Heart," which I pantomimed with deeply felt, full-throttle energy—gripping a bottle of Jack Daniel's or Southern Comfort as a proxy microphone, occasionally letting out a loud, ferocious cackle. The more I learned about Joplin's short, sad life, the more reasons I had to relate to her—and to feel anxious and uncomfortable with that. Janis never thought she fit in either and wasn't such a hit with the hippie boys herself. Shy and artistic by nature, in public she was messy, loud, and arguably androgynous. I already felt like I was all of those things and didn't want to cultivate them further.

I DROPPED OUT of high school to go on Dead tour effectively full-time and became especially close to three other girls. One was very much in the Botticelli mode, having emerged from her suburban New York half shell with bright blue eyes, a dusting of freckles across her cheeks and tiny nose, and perfectly blond, silky hair. We briefly shared the attentions of the same tour-head bro, a tall and charming and popular drug dealer. One night, he and I sat smoking a joint and talking on a little patch of spare dry grass in the parking lot of the arena the Dead had just played in, in North Carolina. He kissed me and ran a hand through my hair. I could tell he was disappointed by how quickly his hand traveled from my scalp to my hair's ends. He shook his head and smiled at me apologetically. "You're a cool girl," he said, "but Marla's so cute." I don't know if this is what precipitated the dissolution of my friendship with Marla. I'm sure it contributed to it. But on tour I remained close to the two other girls. One, Teri, was Native American, with very dark, sometimes unruly hair. The other, Wendi, was half-Indonesian, with the thickest, blackest, and most exquisite hair I'd ever seen. Teri and Wendi were both beautiful, but not in the conventional hippie-girl way. I felt safe and secure in their sisterly company.

When hair wraps became all the rage on tour—most of us Deadhead girls bound a few hanks of our hair with multicolored embroidery floss and sometimes finished them with a flourish of beads—they felt like a blessing: a way of controlling and taming my hair, fully sanctioned and embraced by my community. I still have a photograph of myself with one of those wraps, but now I can see that I was fooling myself. If anything, it made the staticky frazzle of the hair that surrounded it really stand out.

IN MY SOPHOMORE year of college—this was a few years after I'd left tour and gotten a GED—I had no recourse one night but to cut off most of my hair after a foolish, failed dreadlock experiment. Instead of neatly partitioned, tight, graceful locks, I'd managed to give myself two massive, knotted, knobby antennae, so cumbersome that I could not find a comfortable way to rest my head on a pillow. That late-night haircut, generated by frustration and fueled by cheap beer and a few shots of whiskey, still stands as the best I've ever had. Released, my curls looked springy and healthy. By accident, I'd created a shape that framed my face just right. I never got more compliments on my hair.

*My hair can only stand to grow so much, and then, when it has no more will, it stops.*

But that cut could never be duplicated, not even by professionals. It was like the Brigadoon of haircuts, a supernatural occurrence that could happen only once in a lifetime.

Still, I kept my hair short, or shortish anyway, for most of my twenties and thirties. It was easy to wash and shake dry with a towel, then fluff up a bit with some gooey curl cream and go. It felt respectable and professional enough for a young woman trying to prove that she was a respectable, professional grown-up, so naturally it never felt like me.

In my early forties, I made what felt like a momentous decision: unless extreme and unusual circumstances (a funeral? an improbable black-tie event? the Kentucky Derby?) forced me to do otherwise, I would never again wear anything that would look out of place on a Fairport Convention or Incredible String Band album cover. (If only I'd paid more attention to those

English folky counterculture types when I was a teenager; they didn't seem to make as much of a fuss over their hair as their American counterparts.) My hair still doesn't want to be long, or straight, or smooth, but I don't think I'll ever really cut it again. Instead, I'll just trim the split ends off every few months. Now that it's perfectly obvious that I am an adult, the pressure to look like one is off. Most days I plait my hair into two braids and pin them up symmetrically, one on each side of my head. My hair may have failed me when I was a hippie girl, but now that I'm a middle-aged hippie woman, it's doing just fine.

# Romance and Ritual

. . . . . . . . . . . . . . . . . . . . . . . . . . . . . . . . . . . . . . . . . . .

## BHARATI MUKHERJEE

As a child growing up in Calcutta in a traditional Hindu Bengali extended-family household, in which all adult women (except my widowed grandmother) and all girl cousins had long, strong, glossy black hair, I developed an unhappy relationship with my own fine, wispy hair. My iron-willed grandmother, who had been born in the nineteenth century, insisted on the family's following the unbending rules of social comportment laid down in the ancient text *The Manusmriti*, circa 1500 BCE, popularly referred to as the Laws of Manu and ascribed to Manu, the First Man. Manu the Lawgiver dictated incontrovertible dos and don'ts on all aspects of Hindu domestic life, including the type and quantity of body hair and head hair desirable in women. Decent men were to avoid women with hairy bodies, women with reddish hair, and women with bald or balding scalps. To ensure the growth of thick hair, girl children in our community have their heads shaved around age four or five in the belief that the second, permanent growth will be stronger and fuller. I too had my head shaved as a young child, but my follicles did not produce thicker, blacker hair.

*Decent men were to avoid women with hairy bodies, women with reddish hair, and women with bald or balding scalps.*

My mother expended a great deal of energy every morning, massaging hair oil into my scalp to increase blood circulation and revive fatigued follicles. This was a prebath ritual. She would sit on a chair, with me squirming on a low stool in front of her, and she would part my locks, strand by strand, in order to work pink hibiscus-scented oil into the follicles. Sometimes she switched to green amla-fruit oil, not only because eating the tart amla fruit, with its sweet aftertaste, was known to control rheumatoid arthritis and osteoporosis, increase intelligence, and improve eyesight, but because the oil processed from it fostered hair growth. In addition, she was always on the lookout for the harder-to-find hair oil pressed from a berry called *koonch* in Bangla, because it was guaranteed to grow new hair. Every two weeks, a half hour before she shampooed my hair, she would slather homemade yogurt on my head to guard against dandruff.

I, an ingrate daughter, resented every aspect of her hair-enhancement rituals, especially having to sacrifice precious leisure time when I would rather have read novels. But now the very memory of my mother's nurturing fingers kneading the oiled-slippery skin on my head, her favorite fine-tooth comb sliding and smoothing tangles, the gentle press of her knees as they supported my slack-muscled bookworm's back, brings on surges of guilt and pleasure. As an adult, I have treated myself to head massages in upscale hotel spas in China, Malaysia, Thailand, and Indonesia. But as a child, given my scanty, secondhand knowledge of Manu the Lawgiver's definitions of ideal hair, I was convinced that my thin hair was a symptom of moral flaws.

The oldest girl cousin in our large household, a know-it-all teenager, had a practical explanation for why Hindu Bengali women were required to have thick, waist-length hair. She was eight or ten years older than I was; I can't be sure. Even though my generation was the first in our family to have been born in a hospital rather than delivered by a midwife at home, we did not have birth certificates. No one in our comfortably middle-class neighborhood did. The dates of individual births and deaths were associated with natural events, such as earthquakes and fatal floods, or with historical and political events, for example, a massive-scale, British Raj–engineered famine in the early 1940s and hangings of nationalist freedom fighters. This cousin informed us younger ones that an essential rite in Hindu Bengali weddings—the wedding ceremony lasts several days—involves the brides washing the feet of her bridegroom and drying his feet with her hair. She herself had coal-black hair, long enough and tough enough to towel-dry the largest, wettest pair of spousal feet. She also confided that if a woman had reddish or brownish hair instead of black, it was inescapable proof that some ancestor of that woman had—horror of horrors!—mated with a *firangi*, a white-skinned foreigner, in the pre–British Raj past when European pirates regularly raided our bountiful coastal towns. Hindu society was divided into distinct castes: maintenance of caste "purity" and vigilant avoidance of caste "pollution" were required of each individual. My family belonged to the Brahmin caste and could marry only within that caste. Neither my cousin nor I had a way of foretelling that at age twenty-three, while a graduate student in the Writers' Workshop at the University of Iowa, I would marry a blue-eyed American fellow student and become the first in my family to commit caste "pollution." Perhaps my opinionated cousin was correct: my husband and I have two sons, and both have brown hair.

The girl children on our block, including my cousins and my two sisters, had healthier relationships with their hair than I had with mine. My sisters inherited my father's thick, curly hair. Curly hair was admired. I had wavy hair, but the longer it grew, the less wavy it was. All of us parted our hair on one side or the other of our heads, preferably alternating sides to ensure the hair part remained narrow. The first time we expected to part our hair in the center would be on our wedding day during the *sindur*-application rite, when the bridegroom rubs lavish quantities of vermilion powder on the center part of his bride. The vermilion red in a Hindu Bengali woman's hair part is the sign that she is married and that her husband is still living. The red represents life force. A married woman must wear *sindur* every day of her married life. The *sindur* containers on the dressing tables of my mother and aunts were intricate artifacts made of silver or polished buffalo horn. Though I have never worn *sindur*, I have collected these containers as homage to the anonymous craftsmen who elevated the functional to the beautiful. The vermilion used by my mother's generation was later discovered by scientists to be cinnabar, containing mercury sulfide. Contemporary women have replaced the toxic original with a harmless vermilion-red powder. Hindu traditions survive by being adaptable.

> *Hindu Bengali tradition requires widows to keep their heads permanently shaved as one of many gestures of penance.*

Unmarried girls and wives take guiltless pride in their long, lustrous hair. But Hindu Bengali tradition requires widows to keep their heads permanently shaved as one of many gestures of penance. My grandmother was the only widow in the household of my Calcutta childhood. I remember the neighborhood itinerant barber, who tended to male customers under a shady tree on the sidewalk, coming to our home to razor-scrape my grandmother's head every week. My fine-boned grandmother actually looked elegant even when, between the barber's trips, her scalp sprouted silvery stubble.

My mother's attempts to improve the quality of hair I had been born with paled in comparison to those of the more competitive mothers of unmarried girls in our neighborhood. Every weekday afternoon after we'd returned from school by bus or rickshaw and hurried through snacks at home, we congregated in the large front yard of the girl who lived next door to me to play until dusk. My sisters and I braided our hair with pretty satin or taffeta ribbons and looped the two braids like hoop earrings, using the ends of the ribbons to anchor them behind each ear. I loved my collection of ribbons, which I stored in cans that had originally contained imported chocolates. My worry was that during energetic games of hide-and-seek, the ribbons would slip off my skinny braids, which would be humiliating enough, and be lost, which would have been tragic. The girls who were obsessed with hair protection wrapped their braids tightly with ugly, black cotton tapes to protect them from sun damage and dust during playtime. At bedtime, they probably rewrapped their braids with clean cotton ribbons so that heads tossing against pillowcases wouldn't result in split ends. My oldest girl cousin was the only one in our family to wrap her braids during the day. On the nights she suffered from what she called "growing pains" in her calves, she repurposed the black ribbons to neutralize the pain by winding them tightly around her legs.

The first wedding of a Mukherjee relative I witnessed, that of a paternal uncle, took place when I must have been five or six. Marriages were "arranged" by family elders on the basis of economic and social compatibility, the groom's career potential, the bride's physical comeliness and fair complexion, and the spousal candidates' families' medical histories (which had to be free of heritable and communicable diseases). The groom was a tall (at least by our standards), handsome young man with a full head of fastidiously groomed, wavy hair. Hindu weddings are elaborate, some ceremonies having to be performed in the bride's home, and a lesser number in the groom's. I remember with astonishing vividness my uncle, dressed in the Bengali bridegroom's fine *dhoti*, silk *kurta*, and tall wedding head gear, ushering his bride in through the

*My sisters and I braided our hair with pretty satin or taffeta ribbons and looped the two braids like hoop earrings, using the ends of the ribbons to anchor them behind each ear. I loved my collection of ribbons.*

front door of our flat as the conch-blowing, ululating women in our family swarmed around her to welcome her. I also remember each adult woman relative sticking honey-dipped fingers into the bride's ears and mouth so that she would hear and utter only sweet words. The literal and the symbolic merge in Hindu rituals, and though I didn't recognize it then, I was learning a lesson useful for my future as a writer. During the wedding rites performed on the day after her arrival in our home, I recall witnessing this new aunt cooking and feeding her bridegroom rice and curried fish, giving him the whole fish's prized head and torso, and keeping (as tradition demanded) the bony tail for herself. Did she wash the bridegroom's feet and dry them with her hair before that ritual meal? I witnessed this ritual act of wifely obeisance, didn't I? I can no longer be sure. A dear New York–based friend of mine, a naturalized US citizen, confided to me that she knew her first marriage was over when, on an impulse, she went to a salon and asked for her long hair to be chopped off. She wears her hair short and is happily remarried.

In the winter of 1948, after India had been a sovereign nation for nearly a year and a half, my father, mother, and we three sisters sailed for Europe, my youngest sister wearing a scarf over her recently shaved head. My father would work for a few years with pharmaceutical companies in Switzerland and England. We returned to Calcutta, but not to the extended-family household with its oppressive allegiance to ancient traditions. We began life as a nuclear family, and I found myself no longer fretting about my fine hair.

I now live in two cities: New York and San Francisco. When I first moved to San Francisco, I felt lucky to have been befriended by a California-born neighbor, who knew the answers to all the settling-in questions that I hadn't yet thought to ask: for example, where to find the freshest fish, the most inspired florist, the masseuse with magic fingers, the caring yoga instructor. The only question that stumped her was where I should go to get a decent, reasonable haircut. It seemed that my hair needs were too simple—a cut, shampoo, and blow-dry every three or four months—for her to send me to the stylists and colorists she patronized. My hair has remained dark, as was my father's hair when he passed away at age seventy-five.

I know my hair is thinning. When I run into old friends visiting the United States from Calcutta, some will exclaim, with the shocking frankness that only Indian friends you have grown up with can, "Bharati, you're getting bald! Good grief, what happened!" There is a medical explanation: recently I've been diagnosed with rheumatoid arthritis, and the medications I have been put on list "loss of hair" as a likely side effect. Maybe I should go back to using amla hair oil, which is said to control rheumatoid arthritis. Maybe I should get a wig. I mentioned the wig idea to Amy Tan over an Italian dinner in Sausalito the night before she was to leave for New York to launch *The Valley of Amazement*, her most recent novel. We've known each other for over twenty years, and she has always come up with suggestions for coping, no matter the nature of the distress. She mailed me a human-hair wig within weeks of that dinner. The hair is lustrous, shoulder length. I take the wig out of the box it came in and caress the silky, supple strands. Apparently, the wig will have to be cut and styled to suit me. Amy has promised to help me find the right stylists. For every problem, there's a solution. I am ready for the next phase of this hair tale: exciting wig adventures with the help of a good friend.

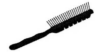

# My Thick Hair

EMMA GILBEY KELLER

**M**y current hairstyle is a shaggy bob. I take it quite seriously. Seriously enough to have a board on Pinterest called "Shaggy Bob," where I add pictures of versions I like. For some reason the board has quite a few followers. They're not my followers (I have loads of boards that are completely ignored) but Shaggy Bob's, so I guess I'm not alone out there in liking this particular style.

What's a shaggy bob? A bob is the neat haircut ending somewhere between ear, chin, and collarbone (think Coco Chanel, Anna Wintour, and various Hillary Clintons), and a shaggy bob is the same thing with layers cut into it for "texture." You might think of this as a scruffy rather than a shaggy bob, but for those of us with a lot of hair, it's the difference between a pyramid shaped wedge (scruffy) and a style that can actually be quite chic (shaggy).

I take my bob seriously enough to get it cut at Sally Hershberger Downtown (but not by Sally Hershberger herself—that would be overdoing it). Sally was the hairdresser who cut the Meg Ryan version of the shaggy bob that became all the rage back in the day. It's the nineties hair of *When Harry Met Sally* and *You've Got Mail*. Goodness, that's over twenty years ago now and Sally's still going strong. I don't want to boast (or age myself more than I have to), but I was getting shaggy bobs in Tribeca as a twentysomething in the late eighties when I first moved to New York from London—for free, by students on certain Saturday mornings at edgy downtown salons on West Broadway.

*"Your hair is so thick," my grandmother used to tell me with a curled-lip emphasis that immediately turned the statement into an insult.*

These days, James at Sally H. cuts my hair. Two good things about him: (1) He can cut the best shaggy bob on the planet. (2) He's a Brit. So when I'm getting my hair done, we talk about the King's Road and hot chocolate and Marmite and all the other things Brits talk about when they're in the USA. The other day, when I was in the salon getting my hair cut, Sally was there too. She works off to one side behind a partition so you can't see her. I knew she was there, though, because they were playing Sally music, Burt Bacharach, instead of whatever they normally play that I never recognize because I'm too old. At that precise moment, I thought I was in heaven. A Brit-cut shaggy bob in New York and Burt Bacharach music. That is so *me*, I thought. This is so *right*.

I HAVE A lot of hair, it's very thick, and it's a good texture. I'll be honest: it's one of my best features, but I wasn't brought up to think of it like that—English people are excellent are turning assets into flaws. And they don't like anything that smacks of wretched excess.

"Your hair is so *thick*," my grandmother used to tell me with a curled-lip emphasis that immediately turned the statement into an insult. Even now I apologize when anyone washing, cutting, or drying it comments on its thickness. "But it's a good thing," they often reply, in surprise. This is one of the reasons I love America.

When I was a child in London, my American mother took my two brothers and me to get our hair cut in the children's department at Harrods, because Harrods was at the end of our street. We loved going there. In the center of the floor was a rocking horse that you could ride when the old ladies had finished their work on your head. No, they didn't put a bowl over the top and cut round it, as legend has it. But looking back at childhood pictures, I can see how that legend got started.

As far as I can remember, they could do only one style, or maybe my mother got a discount for getting three haircuts all the same. Still, my brothers and I came out all looking identical. If I asked about this, I was told I needed to keep my hair that short because it was so . . . thick. When I got to an age to mildly rebel—I was ten—I asked if I could grow my hair. I was told that because of its thickness it simply couldn't grow past my shoulders. Thickness, as I remember it, was presented to me as a disability. I remember the conversations like this:

ME: Can I have my hair a bit longer?
MY MOTHER: No, it's too thick.
ME: But it's so short.
MY MOTHER: Because it's so thick. (*Walks off.*)
ME: (*Rolls eyes.*)

Now I realize she meant it was too thick to be long, because it would look messy. Someone—my mother, for instance—would have to brush it. I can see how all of that seemed like too much effort. Life was an enormous effort for my mother when I was a child. Laundry, grocery shopping, housework, even hair brushing, were either farmed out to other people or just not done. So I accepted a compromise, happy not to look like a boy as I was allowed to grow my hair just as far as my ears. That's how I got my first little bob.

I had a fringe too. Or what Americans called bangs. This

was because my eyebrows weren't round like most people's but went up into little mountain peaks at the center. I was called Spock at school. Until I got the fringe. Then the eyebrows were thankfully obscured and everyone shut up.

My mother had a sense of humor that I found incomprehensible as a child but am more in tune with now that I have daughters of my own. On my first passport application, when I was some tender age under five, she wrote "auburn" for hair color, and they accepted it. "Eyes: green. Hair: auburn." And so it continued through each passport renewal until I was an adult. My mother was living in a society she had a love-hate relationship

*Life was an enormous effort for my mother when I was a child. Laundry, grocery shopping, housework, even hair brushing, were either farmed out to other people or just not done.*

with. The school uniforms and convent boarding school of my childhood were part of her hate. But with "Eyes: green. Hair: auburn," she showed me how to be subversive—and glamorous. Until one day when the passport system caught on to the joke, and my hair officially turned brown.

It's still brown auburn, but no longer naturally. My two daughters have inherited my hair, so I can see the original on them. I have the expensive auburn highlights that women my age graduate to when time and circumstances go our way. We call them "caramel" and "honey." We use the words "tawny" and "ash." In the summer, we can go as far as "buttery," but we have to be careful. We don't want to look cheap.

The highlights cost a fortune, but I can't tell you the exact amount, as I've taught myself not to look when I sign the credit card slip. The tips alone make me blush. I like to tell people I have the most expensive hair in New York, but I know I'm wrong. Those women sitting behind Sally H.'s partition are certain to have bills higher than mine.

When I was pregnant with my first child, Molly, I didn't cut my hair. I felt like Björn Borg, who never cut his hair or shaved during Wimbledon, for luck. My hair grew and grew, finally long, and thicker than ever, due to pregnancy hormones and prenatal vitamins. I loved it. Then Molly was born, a large, bouncy, overdue baby. Everything was there—except hair. She was completely bald until she was two. Whose joke was that?

I kept my hair long throughout Molly's early years and those of her younger sister, Alice. The Spock eyebrows were professionally dealt with on a monthly basis so I could get rid of the bangs. I got my hair blown out once a week, and I turned into a sleek New York City housewife. My English friends described me as "glossy" with that same age-old inflection I understood not to be complimentary. Then the girls grew older, and their hair grew longer. It grew down their backs and it was beautiful. It made mine look like what it was, the older woman's version of long, thick hair. Time for a haircut—a return to the shaggy bob.

Coincidentally, my decision to return to the hairstyle of my youth occurred just before I was diagnosed with breast cancer. Was I aware of the coincidence? I'd say not. Instead I'd point out that most breast cancer diagnoses come in late middle age, and that's when most women change hairstyles anyway. What I will admit to is a multitude of visits to the hairdresser before, during, and after my bilateral mastectomy. My body looked awful—swollen, misshapen, and scarred. But if you looked at my

*When I was pregnant with my first child, Molly, I didn't cut my hair. I felt like Björn Borg, who never cut his hair or shaved during Wimbledon, for luck.*

hair, you'd think nothing was wrong. A week after my operation, my surgeon told me I was done. No chemo or radiation in my future, because surgery had removed the cancer in its early entirety. The relief at not having to have chemotherapy was enormous, but as I recall I never once considered losing my hair. I just assumed there was so much of it, it would somehow survive.

I found it soothing to get my hair done while I recovered from surgery. A beauty salon was the antithesis of a doctor's office. It was a place I could relax and emerge looking better. Looking better made me feel healthier. It lifted my spirits.

Later that same year, my father died. I spent the last week of his life with him in hospital on the British East Anglian coast. I was in his room practically round the clock and loved being there. I did leave one lunchtime to go to a local place for a wash and blow-dry, but I hated the experience and the result. It was the wrong time to look for an escape. After my dad died, I got on the train to London and went straight to get my hair cut very short. It was similar to my first little ear-length bob.

I've often read about women getting trauma cuts. This was mine. My grief at my father's death was enormous. I was completely engulfed by it. My bob cut back to my ears was its sign. The contrast strikes me now as I write about it. Long, long hair at the birth of my daughter; short, short hair at the death of my father.

Some women might extend the comparison and say something along the lines of there being a reason I was born with thick hair. It's a reflection of the richness of my life and so on. But I'm afraid that's not my style. Still, it's made me think about a period in my early thirties when I drove a convertible VW with the roof permanently down. I felt very Italian. My love life was a chaos that I remember as a series of unfortunate events. My hair was one big tangled mess. That's the analogy for me.

What shall I do with my hair as I grow old? Recently I went to Sweden, where the population is homogeneous enough to describe in broad strokes. I looked at the hair of women in their fifties and sixties and was thrilled to see that they all had shaggy bobs! True, some of them were shaggier than others, and some had bangs while others didn't. But the bobs were there, blond and heavily highlighted. No need to go gray, it seems. Yet the faces were bare of makeup and free from cosmetic procedures. It's a pretty look. Still scruffy but still chic. Feminine, with a definite toughness. This is the hairstyle I want as an old woman. This is how I see myself aging. With thick auburnish hair and wise, green eyes. Glamorous and subversive—still living as my mother taught me to be.

# Oh Capello

. . . . . . . . . . . . . . . . . . . . . . . . . . . . . . . . . . . . . . . . . . . . . .

ADRIANA TRIGIANI

*Let me take you back in time to a garden in Pompeii, Italy, in AD 79-ish.*

*Imagine an Italian mother and her daughter. Pretend it's my mom and me. My mother has perfect Dolores del Rio/Hedy Lamarr hair; present day, think Penélope Cruz and Shalom Harlow, hairwise. Think smooth, full, waxy, straight brunette hair. For the daughter, imagine Lionel Richie's full-moon Afro from his early days with the Commodores.*

*There, beneath the hot Italian sun somewhere outside Rome and just a few kilometers from Naples, Mother sits in her garden sorting beans, her raven hair in a sleek chignon, while her daughter, her unruly hair slicked back with a rope, helps. Lava begins to pour from Vesuvius. Sounds of running and screaming, while molten goo spews over the village. Mother looks at daughter. Instead of saying "Run!" she says, "I wish we could do something with your hair."*

I CAME UP in the age of Madonna Ciccone, a pop star who changed her hair daily. It was so much fun to watch her go from pitch-black geisha to mahogany-brown curls, from a dirty-blond pixie to neutron-blond bob. But once she hit her midforties, she went Upper East Side blond, where she has stayed for about twelve years. This is upsetting to me, as I expect trends out of her, not long hair with split ends snipped at Supercuts, like, say, my own hair. I figure when Madonna gets scared about changing her hair, something is about to blow again, like Vesuvius.

*I figure when Madonna gets scared about changing her hair, something is about to blow again, like Vesuvius.*

I watch TCM a lot and study the movie stars of the golden age of Hollywood for hair inspiration. I've had every hair incarnation from the sculptured medium-length hair of Myrna Loy to the sassy short cut of Jean Simmons in the Bible epic, but no matter what I do, my curls fight their way through, and I'm right back at Shirley Temple. Luckily, she gets a film festival once a year on TCM.

I come from a big family. Most of the kids in the family

have my mother's hair, a sleek brunette version of wavy, bordering on straight. I got my father's hair, tight curls and fine texture, as if B. B. King and Louis Prima had a baby. The tight curls were there when I was an infant, and then they sort of shook out until I was a teenager, when they came roaring back just in time to kill any chance I might be asked out on a date. Never one to sulk, I shook up my routine and cut my long hair short, into a wedge. It was a disaster. I was the only girl in my ninth-grade class who looked fifty-three.

It wasn't that I was unsophisticated. Yes, I was growing up in the glorious Blue Ridge Mountains, but I read fashion magazines, went to the library, and even bought an out-of-print beauty book from the fifties, a primer called *Taffy's Tips to Teens*. There was a section that helped the reader figure out her face shape so she could choose a complementary hairdo. Taffy instructed the reader to stand in front of a mirror and outline her face with a crayon on the glass. You figured out your shape: oblong, oval, square, round, or heart shaped (mine was a shape called old sponge).

According to Taffy (surely a nom de plume for a drunk book editor out to make extra money to go on a cruise), you were to

> *Never one to sulk, I shook up my routine and cut my long hair short, into a wedge. It was a disaster. I was the only girl in my ninth-grade class who looked fifty-three.*

choose the hairstyle that went with your face shape and stick to it for life. Taffy said I was never to get a pixie. I was never to get a chin-length bob. She didn't mention the wedge, so I figured I was safe. In retrospect, it may be that it was the combination of the short cut and the ashtray-thick lenses in my eyeglasses that ruined my social life, but we can never be sure. All I know is that Taffy's hair rules have stuck. To this day, when I see a long-faced woman with a slicked-back bun, I think, Forehead alert: Taffy said no. You need bangs. *Bangs!*

Taffy said a good hairdresser was as important as a good doctor.

I went on a lifelong search to find someone who could cut my hair properly. I did not find that person in Virginia or Indiana. I had high hopes when I moved to New York City, because there was a hair salon on every corner. Surely the odds were finally in my favor and one of these folks could do the job. I learned one important lesson as I went from salon to salon. Never trust a salon with three names if all of them are first names. I could get a good cut at the Gloria In Excelsis Deo Salon, but never at the Charles Thomas William Salon.

I've gone to fancy beauty parlors, low-rent salons, and, once, a woman's basement in Queens in order to save fifty bucks, but it was a wash, since I ended up spending the cash I saved on a cab because I was late for the train. Avoid any long-distance travel when it comes to hair—always choose your neighborhood over a long drive or train ride or flight. If you make it impossible for yourself geographically, you'll be one of those people who is forever letting a cut "grow out." When you look up "grow out a cut" in the beauty bible, it translates to "cheap and lazy" or "you deserve whatever happens to you because you went to a basement in Queens."

I'm not blaming the stylists for letting me down. When you have curly hair, your choice in cut is somewhere between Barbra Streisand in *A Star Is Born* and Barbra Streisand in *The Main Event*. Stylists try so hard to change up curly hair, but there are really only two techniques: they either blunt-cut it or layer it. That's all. You could use nail scissors or a Weedwacker, but the results will pretty much be the same—unless you cut bangs. Then you have the Mamie Eisenhower problem.

Mamie, the First Lady of the 1950s, had a wave in her hair, therefore her bangs had a crimp. You don't want crimps in your bangs; you want them to lie flat like the fringe on an ottoman. Every once in a while, I forget this rule, cut the bangs, and have to blow them straight. I get so tired doing this chore, I leave the rest curly—which gives me the look of a stern poodle or a beauty slacker who was exhausted and decided to blow only the front of her head.

Hair is so important to people. When I wrote for television, I couldn't believe how critical hair was to final casting decisions. Long hair was the only way to go for women—even if they were over eighty. Men had to have hair, store bought or otherwise, even if they were over eighty.

I would study the faces of the actors at auditions, listen to their words, and watch as a character on the page seemed to inhabit their bodies as they interpreted a scene. The network saw nothing but hair. "But we can change the hair!" I'd proclaim. They would look at me as though mine were on fire.

Why couldn't executives imagine a sultry brunette as a hot blond, or a hot blond as a glorious redhead? Perhaps my curls made me think outside the box. I acknowledge the possibilities of hair because my own is so limiting. I refused to accept that hair alone could kill any chance an actor had at a great role. I was so relieved that a writer didn't have to obsess about such things, though more than one person has told me that behind my back, producers would say, "Get me that curly-haired Italian girl in New York."

No one escapes the hair label.

I married a man with hair, and now I'm married to a man who only has some. Same guy. Is it a sin that I love that he's bald? My husband is handsome, but without hair he looks older than me, which is the great blessing of a long marriage. One day a man came to fix our furnace, and he said, "The last time I was here, I told your father this furnace was on borrowed time." I didn't bother to tell the repairman that my father had been dead for nine years. Instead, I left him there and tore up those rickety basement stairs to call my husband. On the way, I fell, hit my chin, bruised my hip, and busted my lip, but it didn't matter. I crawled to the phone to tell my husband the bad news: We need a new furnace. And the good news: The repairman thinks you're my father!

When I get depressed, I just think of that story, and suddenly I'm gay and happy and it's springtime everywhere!

When I had a baby girl with my handsome husband, I was shocked when her hair grew in—it was blond—and it was straight. When I took her to the park, people spoke Spanish to me. With my dark hair, they thought I was her nanny. The mix-up was not without its benefits. I learned that "arriba" on the swings means "Push me higher, Mommy!"

Any conversation about hair is really, at its root, about vanity. I learned that early on, as a theater major in college, when one of my first jobs was to dye an actor's brown hair gray. I read the instructions on the box carefully, but as a brunette, I knew very little about peroxide. I applied the creamy mixture to the actor's hair and put a shower cap on his head. When I removed the cap about forty minutes later, his hair was the color of a new lime—a bright yellowish green. The director began to scream; the actor, to weep. The look in the young man's eyes when he saw that I had turned him into something you shove into a Bloody Mary was one I will never forget. The director ran around in a circle like Henny Penny, cursing me. I had ruined their lives; at the very least, their play. But I didn't let it kill my spirit. When you entrust your head to a girl with 20/80 vision in one eye and an astigmatism and 20/200 in the other, you get what you pay for, which, for the record, was green hair.

Flash forward to last year, when I found Edward, the perfect stylist, after a lifetime of searching for him. Our enchantment was mutual and immediate. When I said, "No soccer mom," he did his best to give me courant and funky with his magic scissors. He was so flexible! I'd call Edward on a whim and he'd take me, any day, any time. The salon where he worked was bohemian in that artistic East Village style. There were mannequins with eyes missing, paintings that moved, and a nude statue that took me four visits to figure out was a nude. The manager, who had to be a great-nephew of Ernest Borgnine, as he was his dead ringer, was six feet three inches and wore kneesocks, culottes, and a Glenda Jackson ginger-red pageboy.

Despite the *House of Wax* decor at the House of Hair, I ignored the surroundings and settled in with Edward. We talked and laughed, and he gave my curls something they hadn't seen in twenty years of growth: he gave them love.

Things could go wrong in my life, and there Edward would be, my stylist and prince, waiting for me with a cold glass of water that had slices of cucumber floating in it (it's good for the hair or the colon; either way, I'm a taker), and I'd relax, knowing that in an hour, I'd have big, wild, shiny curls, fashion be ignored and be damned, in an era where even Lionel Richie has straight hair.

Edward would tell me that he loved my curls, and his enthusiasm made me love them too. In an age where every third person asks me if I've "tried a blowout" or tells me "you should do keratin," I realize that this straight-hair-over-curly thing is real: they want curls banned. I'm a rebel—well, not exactly. I just do what's easy—and *easy* translated from the Italian means curly (and if it doesn't, it should).

One day, Edward called me. He said he had to leave New York City. He had seen a news report that said if everyone left their apartments in Manhattan at the same moment, the population of the city could not fit in the streets. He couldn't live in a place where everyone couldn't fit in the streets and he hoped I understood. He said he was going to find himself. I said, "Edward, if you are going to find yourself, who was that man who gave me the perfect haircut?" He laughed and told me that life is short. Hair grows out, and people have to grow up. He called this his *Eat, Pray, Love* tour. He told me he needed to see the world in a new way. Evidently my curls could not make him stay. I wished him well, hung up, and had a nervous breakdown.

I called my mother and told her about Edward's soul-journ. She was silent as I wept. Finally she said, "Now, will you try a blowout? Curls are out, you know."

I know, Ma. I know.

# Why Mothers and Daughters
# Tangle over Hair

## DEBORAH TANNEN

"**D**o you like your hair that long?" my mother asked, soon after I arrived for a visit. I laughed. Looking slightly hurt, she asked why I was laughing. "I've been interviewing women for the book I'm writing about mothers and daughters," I explained, "and so many tell me that their mothers criticize their hair." "I wasn't criticizing," my mother said, and I let it drop. Later in my visit I asked, "So Mom, what do you think of my hair?" Without missing a beat, she replied, "I think it's a little too long."

I wasn't surprised by any of this, because my mother always thought my hair was too long. I'd taken to getting a haircut shortly before visiting my parents, sometimes the very morning before I boarded a plane to Florida. But that never made a difference. I could count on her telling me my hair was too long.

While talking to women for the book *You're Wearing THAT?: Understanding Mothers and Daughters in Conversation*, I collected a cornucopia of mothers' remarks on their daughters' hair. Many of these comments were more overtly critical than my mother's, such as "Comb your hair. The birds will make a nest in it." Some were both overt and indirect: "You did that on purpose?" Sometimes the wolf of criticism came dressed in the sheep's clothing of a compliment: "I love your hair when it's pushed back off your face," said when her daughter's hair was falling forward onto her face, or "I'm so glad you're not wearing your hair in that frumpy way anymore."

*Sometimes it wasn't criticism that frustrated women so much as the focus on hair instead of matters the daughters thought more important.*

Sometimes it wasn't criticism that frustrated women so much as the focus on hair instead of matters the daughters thought more important. During a presidential campaign season, a journalist interviewed both candidates for president. When her mother asked, "How did it go?" she began an enthusiastic account of the interviews. "No," her mother interrupted, "I mean at the hair salon. What style did you settle on? Did you put it up or leave it down?" Another woman told me that after she appeared on television standing behind the president of the United States in a bill-signing ceremony, her mother's comment was, "I could see you didn't have time to cut your bangs."

I came to think of the subjects about which mothers (and daughters) were critical as the big three: hair, clothes, and weight. I always thought of them in that order, because hair was the subject of the largest number of remarks repeated to me, and, it seemed, the most unnerving.

Why? Why so much preoccupation with hair? I first asked myself this question years ago, while taking part in a small academic conference at which each participant—eight men and four women—gave a brief presentation. As I listened to one of the women give her talk, I was distracted by her hair, which seemed intentionally styled to render her half-blind. When she looked down to read her paper, thanks to a side part and no bangs, a curtain of hair fell clear across her face, completely covering one eye. As she read aloud, she kept reaching up to push the hair off her face, but it immediately fell right

> *Another woman told me that after she appeared on television standing behind the president of the United States in a bill-signing ceremony, her mother's comment was, "I could see you didn't have time to cut your bangs."*

back, a result she ensured by stopping short of hooking it behind her ear. She must have believed that pinning her hair behind her ear would spoil its style.

After catching myself concentrating on the speaker's hair rather than her talk, I scanned the room to check out the other two women's hairstyles. One, the youngest among us, had long frosted blond hair that cascaded over her shoulders—an effect she enhanced by frequently tossing her head. The third woman had dark brown hair in a classic style that, I thought to myself, was a cross between Cleopatra and Plain Jane.

Then I wondered why I was scrutinizing only the women; what about the men? A glance around the room made the answer obvious: every one of the men had his hair cut short, in no particular style. There could have been a man with a ponytail or a thick, wavy mane or long hair falling below his ears. But there wasn't. All the men had chosen neutral hairstyles. What, I asked myself, would be a comparably neutral hairstyle for a woman? Then I realized: there's no such thing.

I came to think of this contrast in terms of a concept from linguistics, my academic field: the men's choices were "unmarked," but any choice a woman makes is "marked"; that is, it says something about her. Here's how linguistic markedness works. The "unmarked" forms of most verbs in English communicate present tense. To communicate past tense, a speaker "marks" a verb by adding something. For example, you can take the verb *visit* and mark it for *past* by adding *-ed* to make *visited*. Similarly, the unmarked forms of most nouns in English are singular, such as *toy*. To make the word plural, you add *–s* to get *toys*. Like a present-tense verb or a singular noun, a man can have a hairstyle that is "unmarked"—that is, neutral; it doesn't tell you anything about him except that he's male. But any choice a woman makes carries extra meaning: it leads observers to conclude something about the type of person she is. That's why I titled an essay on this subject "There Is No Unmarked Woman."

The concept of markedness helps explain many mothers' seemingly excessive concern with so apparently superficial a topic as their daughters' hair. They are thinking of how others will interpret their daughters' character. That concern was explicit in one mother's warning that no one would take her daughter seriously if she didn't style her hair more carefully: "If they see someone with loose ends in their hair, they'll think you have loose ends in your life."

Mothers aren't the only ones who are inclined to be critical of women's hair (as well as their clothes and weight). Because the range of hairstyles from which a woman must choose is so vast, the chances that anyone—especially another woman—will think she made the best choice are pretty slim. How often do you look at a woman and think, She would look better if her hair were . . . longer, shorter, curlier, straighter, pushed back, pulled forward, colored, not colored, dyed a different color, highlighted or not, more fashionably styled, just differently styled? We think these things, but we don't say them. A mother, however, often feels she has a right if not an obligation to say something, because it's her job to ensure that things go as well as possible for her daughter.

There is yet another layer to all of this: women's and girls' hair (as well as clothes and weight)—indeed, the preoccupation with women's appearance more generally—is inextricably intertwined with sex. Our very notion of "woman" entails sexuality in a way that our notion of "man" does not. A woman who is not attractive is dismissed, and being deemed attractive requires being sexy—but not too sexy, because that would lead to her being dismissed in a different way. Furthermore, the line between too sexy and not sexy enough is a fine one and is located differently by different observers, so there is no way a woman can be certain of getting it just right. This criterion drives many, if not all, fashion choices: how short or long a skirt or dress should be; how tight-fitting and shape-showing slacks, tops, or dresses should be; how much skin is revealed, what body parts are glimpsed or displayed. And hair is an essential element in this sexual equation.

Hair, in short, is a secondary sex characteristic: like breasts and the distribution of body fat that gives women a curvy shape, more head hair (and less facial hair) is one of the physical features distinguishing the sexes that begin to appear during puberty, signaling sexual maturity. Enhancing and drawing attention to secondary sex characteristics can be a way of emphasizing sexual attractiveness. Thus, hair so abundant that it partially covers a woman's face can be sexy, and more hair can be sexier than less. That is the aesthetic that drives "big hair," and the anxiety that underlies the concept of a "bad-hair day." And that is the reason why many societies require women to cover, hide, or remove their hair. The connection between exposing hair and seeking to attract men is explicit in the Orthodox Jewish tradition by which women cut off their hair when they marry, as my grandmother did in the early 1900s Hasidic Jewish community of Warsaw. (My father was told that when his mother was having her head shaved in preparation for her wedding, her younger sisters, who had abandoned orthodoxy, pounded on the door, begging her not to let them do it; she later regretted having acquiesced and let it grow back.)

This tradition came to mind when I asked an Arab woman whether mothers in her country comment on their daughters' appearance. She replied that a common mother-to-daughter remonstrance would be, "I can see hair"—a way to admonish a daughter to tighten her head scarf. Though the requirement to wear head scarves might seem at first very different from the "freedom" to expose hair, these seemingly opposite customs are really two sides of the same coin, divergent ways of managing men's responses to this secondary sex characteristic: on one hand, precluding it by hiding hair, on the other capitalizing on it by displaying hair in as alluring a style as possible.

WHILE I WAS working on this essay, my phone rang. It was my cousin Elaine calling. "I'm visiting my mother," she began. I was concerned, because I knew that her mother had recently been discharged from the hospital after a life-threatening illness. Elaine continued, "What do you think was the first thing she asked me?" Still living in this essay, I offered, half-joking, "Was it about your hair?" "Yes!" she exclaimed. "That *is* what she asked! I had been here maybe ten minutes when she said, 'Don't you think you need a haircut?'"

"You won't believe this," I said, and then read her the first paragraph of this essay.

After we both laughed at the uncanny similarity, Elaine continued, "I'm trying to assert myself now that I'm sixty, so I told her, 'I just had it cut!'" She explained that she'd made sure to do that because her mother always thinks her hair is too long. At that I read her the second paragraph of this essay.

After more shared laughter, Elaine resumed her account. Her mother kept returning to the topic: "Are you sure you don't think it would be better shorter?" and "We have to go to my hairdresser." Elaine capitulated: "I was in her house for less than half an hour before she was whisking me off, walker and all, to her hair salon!" But Elaine drew the line at cutting her hair; she submitted only to having it blow-dried. Then she questioned her own sanity when, upon hearing her mother say, "Now you're a pleasure to look at," she heard herself say: "Maybe it would have been better shorter."

After we laughed together, our conversation turned serious. Wondering aloud why her mother's concern with her hair bothered her so much, Elaine said, "It's a symbol of lack of acceptance." Without doubt, that's part of why we all react so strongly to perceived criticism, no matter how subtle, from our mothers—and why many of us are so quick to perceive criticism in any comment or, for that matter, gesture (like reaching out to brush hair off our faces) or facial expression ("I didn't say anything"; "But you had that look"). There is an exquisite irony—a perfect relationship storm, you might say—between daughters and mothers. Because girls and women are judged by appearance, mothers want their daughters to look as attractive as possible. But any suggestion for improvement implies criticism. And therein lies the irony: for mothers, the person to whom you most want to offer helpful suggestions is the one most likely to resist and resent them; for daughters, the person you most want to think you're perfect is the one most likely to see your flaws—and tell you about them.

My cousin then told me something I hadn't known: her mother hated her own hair, because *her* mother had told her it was ugly. Indeed, Elaine's mother had gone to medical school to ensure she'd be able to support herself, because her mother had led her to believe she was too unattractive to count on getting married. How, Elaine wondered, could her mother not see that she was doing to her daughter just what her own mother had done to her? There are many ways to answer that question. One is that Elaine's mother wanted to make sure her daughter *didn't* suffer the same fate, by making sure she *was* attractive. Another is that she was doing what many women do: both mothers and daughters often regard each other as reflections of themselves and consequently look at each other with a level of scrutiny that they otherwise reserve for themselves. For mothers, especially, that isn't entirely irrational: they are held responsible for their daughters in a way that fathers are not. Someone who disapproves of a girl's appearance will often think, Why did her mother let her go out looking like that?

*Someone who disapproves of a girl's appearance will often think, Why did her mother let her go out looking like that?*

Maybe it doesn't matter what mothers' motives are. The challenge for daughters is deciding how to respond. I always chuckle when recalling the woman who told me she silenced her mother by saying, "My lifetime interest in the topic of my hair has been exhausted."

Or perhaps more important than figuring out what to say in response to perceived criticism is how to stop feeling bad about it. Women tell me it helps to realize that criticizing and caring are expressed in the same words. That way, a daughter can shift her focus from the criticizing to the caring. This often happens automatically after our mothers are gone, or when we fear losing them. One woman told me of getting a call that her mother had been hospitalized. Full of worry and fear, she caught a plane and rushed to the hospital right from the airport. Distressed to see her mother with an IV bag attached to her arm and an oxygen tube in her nose, she approached the bedside and leaned over to give her a kiss. Her mother looked up at her and said, "When's the last time you did your roots?" Rather than reacting with her usual annoyance, the daughter heaved a sigh of relief: her mother was OK.

As for me, it is now nearly a decade since my mother died. Several years ago, I began getting my hair cut shorter. My mother was right: it does look better this way.

# Beautiful, Beautiful

. . . . . . . . . . . . . . . . . . . . . . . . . . . . . . . . . . . . . . . . . . . . . . . .

## HONOR MOORE

**T**here is heat at the back of my neck, a spot of heat that gets hotter and hotter. I take the combs out, swirl my hair up, stick the combs in, wear my hair up until my nape cools down. After years of this, I came to understand why women of a certain age cut their hair short, why even the most revolutionary of nineteenth-century feminists acquiesced to the requirements of modesty and wore their hair up. It's hormones! I have been told that the dance of my hands twisting and lifting my thick curtain of hair is an act of kinetic sculpture. Once, when I was in my late forties, a student hit on me: "I couldn't take my eyes off of you, how you kept putting your hair up and taking it down." The kinetic sculpture has by now become a comedy, hair up, hair down, hair up, hair down. And the combs—what a collection I have! Made of plastic by Medusa's Heirlooms, the size of a calling card, ivory, malachite, zebra striped or azure, with teeth that hold. . . . But my subject is my hair, the greatest gift bestowed on me by my ancestors, my gene pool, my biology.

## Lady Godiva

She rode a white horse and she bathed in milk. Her skin was as pale as mine and her hair as dark. It fell to the ground. On that horse she was headed somewhere with her beauty, was how I read the image: somewhere *else*. Her hair was what gave her the beauty that would get her anywhere she wanted to go, out of the suffocating palace, away from the noise, the dirt, the school on the narrow Jersey City avenue, the classroom where none of the books had ladies like Godiva in them, let alone white horses ridden by women. It was in a book that I first saw her, so graceful in her milk bath, outside her window moon and stars that were silver and gold, actual silver and gold gilt on the page. I can't decide whether to google Lady Godiva or not. Why would I want to learn that she was a revolutionary who wore her hair that way for a cause, or that her hair wasn't as long as all that, or that she didn't bathe

> *I have been told that the dance of my hands twisting and lifting my thick curtain of hair is an act of kinetic sculpture.*

in milk, or that she died young. She was Anglo-Saxon, I read, the wife of a nobleman. Legend has it that she protested her husband's taxation of his tenant farmers; he would abolish the tax, he said, if she rode through the town naked. She agreed, on the condition that the populace be confined to their homes so that no one would see her; a man named Tom (the first Peeping Tom) drilled a hole in his window shutters, and when he looked at her he was struck blind. Lady Godiva was widowed fairly young but lived into old age, a devout hermit. (Notice the noun, not usually applied to a woman.) No one has ever been able to find her grave.

## Hard Corners

I was maybe five years old, standing in front of a mirrored door in my grandmother's house in the green hills of New Jersey. It was a very big house with large, high-ceilinged bedrooms, so you could be in your room and feel really alone, even though there were people downstairs or two rooms away. Sometimes my mother came there with us, but more often she didn't, placing her many children for the weekend at our grandmother's, a vacation for her. Without her voice in my ear or her eyes seeing me, I can stand alone and freely look at myself. Finally I have the hair I want. It's just past my shoulders but sure to grow farther down my back.

My mother had short hair then, but in her wedding pictures her black hair is long, shiny, turned under at the ends, in what was called a pageboy. "Your mother should cut her hair," said

Gagy, whose real name was Aagot; she was Norwegian and
often took care of us. My mother had just disappeared into
another room. "Why?" "When you're older, you should not
have hair that long." "But Gagy, your hair is long." "But I
never wear it down." Which was true. I never saw her wear
her hair down, just up, 1940s-style, gathered into coils on either side of her face. I decide I will not give in like my mother
has and cut my hair short or even wear it up like Gagy does.
I will wear it down and long for as long as I want.

I don't remember how I looked so much as how my hair
felt as I ran my hands through it. Soft, long, straight. I do
remember it was lighter brown then, the way brown can look
in a washed-out 1950s Kodachrome. Within weeks of that
moment at the mirror, my mother took me to a hotel in
New York to have my hair cut. She and I had already argued;
we were standing just inside a walk-in closet at my grandmother's when she said, "It's time for you to get a haircut."
We did not fight again at the hairdresser, but I am sure I
wanted to cry.

I believed my hair was how I might claim beauty, and
beauty was freedom I would make for myself, not artifice
designed by others. My mother with her short hair had be-
trayed her beauty; she was always smiling in those photographs with the pageboy, and now she hardly smiled at all.
I wanted to laugh and dream and run free, hair streaming
behind me. When the cut was over, I had bangs; my hair was

short and somehow darker. It stopped just below my ears, and all the softness was gone, along with the honey color I had seen that day in front of the mirror. Now there would be no beauty: I had hard corners.

### Resistance

When I was ten, I got glasses, horn-rims that my mother chose in the spirit of my straight-across bangs and hard-cornered haircut. I was commuting from where we lived in Jersey City to school in Greenwich Village. It was 1955, two years before *On the Road*, but already, at age ten, I had my first pair of black tights. I can't remember if I also wore a black turtleneck, but I had seen people on Bleecker Street who wore black and had very long hair. After the Russians launched Sputnik, they would be called beatniks. I was dressing for the coming era, its advent abruptly interrupted when we moved to Indianapolis two years later. Even madras had not quite arrived in that part of the Midwest; it was still the era of sweater sets, saddle shoes, circle pins, and short, curly hairdos. My hair is very thick but also very fine, which meant that it did not easily hold the wave I set it for in pin curls. I should get a permanent, my mother decided, her solution to my feelings of displacement. I was in seventh grade.

I am trying to resist various metaphors, one of which has my hair as Guatemala and my mother the neo-imperialist secretary of state John Foster Dulles. It works pretty well: I did not have self-determination; she did not believe I knew what was good for me. What I didn't say was that I knew what was good for her. If she would only grow her hair out again, she would understand everything about me and look beautiful again.

*I believed my hair was how I might claim beauty, and beauty was freedom I would make for myself, not artifice designed by others.*

By the time I got to high school, the hair-strafing permanent, which had failed to improve my social life, had grown out. The fashion was to wear your hair even shorter than mine was, in something called a bubble or, depending on I don't know what, a ducktail. A bubble required curlers, which were, by 1960, called rollers. I think of my Hoosier classmate Nancy Peters, whose bubble fluffed into a perfect oval and whose hair was the same color as mine. Betsy Buck, who was blond, had the perfect ducktail: short hair curving around the skull toward the back of the head, swirling up at her nape, and resolving an inch or so higher in a graceful point upward. If I had a bubble like Nancy Peters, I too would be a cheerleader, I reasoned—"popular" and therefore flirted with, dated, and invited to pledge all the good clubs. To become popular, I gave up my secret dream of beauty. I cut my hair, and every time I washed it I rolled a strand over each curler and stuck it through with a plastic stick. When I left for school at 7:30

a.m., my hair was curly, but by the time I got to class, it had always "fallen." In my smiling graduation photograph, my hair is very short and straight and pulled back with a headband that leaves a tiny fringe of bang to soften the expanse of my forehead.

I should say that my mother's hair was naturally wavy, so it wasn't as if she actually understood my straight, fine hair; in any case, by 1959 her hair was very short, and she was pregnant with her eighth child and blessedly distracted from my hair except for an occasional skirmish in the downstairs bathroom. "Get your hair out of your face, sweetie," she would declare, taking a lock between her fingers and guiding it behind my ear. "There, much prettier!" I would refuse and refuse. I didn't want to be pretty. Pretty was ordinary; I wanted to be beautiful and unusual. I wanted to be myself. The battle would escalate, at least once ending with her slapping me, hard, across the face.

## Rivalry

But I have left out an important part of this narrative, which is that my sister, four years younger than I, was always allowed to grow her hair, at least after that square-corners visit to the hairdresser. Why? At first, it was because she was still a "little girl." She wore her hair in pigtails, always. In memory it seems that her hair was not as thick as mine, therefore more easily confined to pigtails. But I would not have wanted to wear braids; my face is round, and I thought they made me look fat. My sister didn't worry about looking fat, since she was smaller boned and therefore thinner than I was; also, the proportions of her face were different from mine and her eyes bigger, so braids suited her. My best friend at the Greenwich Village school was half-Icelandic and wore her hair in long, thick blond braids, which I admired but did not envy. I believe now that I thought my mother favored my sister; why else would she let her grow her hair? Once, when my sister and I discussed my stormy relationship with our mother, she told me that she had observed how I was treated and had done everything she could to avoid getting caught in the line of my mother's fire. She never overate and kept her hair out of her face.

### A President's Wife

I arrived in Cambridge, Massachusetts, as a Radcliffe freshman, in the fall of 1963, the era of Jackie Kennedy. With not much effort, I could make my hair, just short of shoulder length, look like the First Lady's, though in order to look more hip than she, I pierced my ears. By the end of freshman year, I wore contact lenses and had mastered her bouffant. That summer at a wedding, I wore a sleeveless turquoise raw silk dress. "Who's the one who looks like Jackie Kennedy?" someone asked.

When the president died, I let my hair grow. It seemed that everything changed then, including my mother's claim to authority over my hair. Or at least that's what I'm tempted to say. I have a passport photograph taken the summer after my junior year, and my hair is distinctly just below my shoulders, which is where it stayed, more or less, until I became a client of a hairdresser in New York City named George Michael, whose specialty was long hair. I had moved to Manhattan in 1969, and there is a photograph of me from 1972 in a dark blue velvet vintage dress, dancing. My hair is honey-colored in the light and almost to my waist, the longest it ever was.

## Evolution

For decades, I grew my hair and had it cut twice a year to all one length, no layering. I had a friend who declared that look my "trademark" and cautioned me against ever changing it. She herself began to color her hair in her twenties and rarely had the same hairdo or hair color for more than two years in a row. Why did I think she knew more about my hair than I did? Shocking, really, that I allowed another woman to take my mother's place as the authority on my hair. One day in my forties, I decided that my hair made me look like a girl and I wanted to look like a woman. I went to a hairdresser named John Sahag, known as the "revolutionist of dry cutting." He was originally from Lebanon, I learned later, but had trained in Paris, and he cut the hair of movie stars and models. A greyhound napped at the corner of his tranquil Madison Avenue salon. I told him that I wanted to keep my hair long, but . . . "You want something a little different," he said. He suggested a piece cut shorter in the front and "a little layering" and assigned me a stylist named Mayumi, whose black hair fell down her back all the way to her knees. That day, she layered my hair, cutting it to a bit below shoulder length, with shorter pieces in the front—a stealth version of bangs that gave me a few wisps around my face. Layering is a form of thinning, so my hair became less heavy, easier to dry and take care of. It also has a little wave, and weirdly, while straight in the front, it is, underneath a thin, straight top layer, very curly in the back.

## Color

"I am almost sixty, and my hair still stubbornly refuses to go gray," my mother's mother wrote to a longtime friend. When I came across that line, I was barely fifty, had no gray whatsoever, and had never dyed my hair. At first, wisps at the left side of my hairline began to turn; no matter, I told myself, I was on my way to being the next Susan Sontag. A black-haired friend had other ideas. "Soon you'll have to make a decision," she said to me one day. "Go see the colorist at Frederic Fekkai." "Maybe," I said, the familiar wave of stubbornness rising. Ten years later, my hair is still mostly dark, graying along the entire perimeter of my front hairline. Extending a bit into the body of my hair, gray only slightly streaks the darkness, but gracefully, like foam along the edges of a big ocean wave. I get my hair cut twice a year, still by Mayumi at John Sahag, though John died in 2005. "Do I have any gray back there?" I always ask as she lifts and snips, lifts and snips. "No, no! Not yet." She now wears her hair to midback and has let it go gray—elegant silvery streaks through an expanse of Japanese black.

### Philosophy

She is a filmmaker, younger than I am by about thirty years, African American, a near celebrity, gay, very gifted, up-to-the-minute chic. We are sitting at breakfast at an artists' colony when she suggests I shave away a patch of hair above my right ear. This will render me asymmetrical, she explains, and therefore cool, even as cool, she implies, as she is. This out of nowhere: I'm flummoxed. Why would I make such a change? Even when it's dirty or I've resorted to a bed-head look, hardly a day goes by when I don't receive a compliment on my never-colored, near-black, long, thick hair. But she has rendered me speechless, bereft of my usual certainty. "Why?" "You'll like it. A change. Something new!" As if at my age I'd want something that ilk of new! "I don't want anything new," I retort, unable to keep myself from sounding defensive. "You can always let it grow back," she replies. Why does she insist? "I don't think so," I say. "Go ahead," she says. "Don't be scared." Scared? Am I scared? I am never scared! "I'm not SCARED," I reply. "It *will*

grow back," she says, with an even smile, as if I, the queen
of hair, of the endlessly growing mop of silken locks, don't
understand that hair grows. "It will always grow back," she
repeats.

### Shave

On one recent night before sleep, I streamed a video, a movie
set in France during the First World War. At the end of the
film, a girl of about seven meets her father for the first time.
It is 1918, just at the end of the fighting; he is British, a soldier, and he and the girl's French mother had been lovers. He
had not known of this child, but now he does know and is
coming to meet her. He approaches a small country cottage,
a grassy path, everything green. The little girl is coming toward him, the father's point of view. Her hair is light brown,
honey-colored in the light, flowing long down her back.

A week later, I had the following dream. A man I know
who is not a haircutter is snipping away at the short gray hair
of the now dead great poet whose early work inspired me
when I began to write poems. She is sitting calmly, which
makes me extremely anxious, especially when I see that beneath her hair is a shaved patch, the very shaved patch I vi-
sualized when the young woman at the artists' colony made
her recommendation. It's clear to me in the dream that the
man is attempting to cut away the poet's power and that he
doesn't notice the shaved patch. I am aware I have chosen a

different path than my great mentor. My power resides in the length and thickness of my hair, and I will never give it up.

## Blow Dry

Mayumi still cuts my hair—the daughter she was pregnant with when we met is now out of college—but every week, the day I teach my first class, a man named Mike Riz blow-dries my hair. I like thinking that I am of a matrilineage of women who, at a certain age, turn the care of their hair over to others. My mother died at fifty, so who knows if she would have been one of us, but my father's mother had her hair permed, curled, and rinsed blue, and my maternal grandmother, the one whose hair stayed brown into her sixties, kept it dyed that color until she went into a nursing home at eighty-five. My immediate predecessors are two aunts, my mother's and father's sisters, who lived near each other and shared only a love of gardening, but ran into each other at the hairdresser once a week. Have I turned into an old lady? I choose to think not. I continue to want the compliments I've received all my life, even from young women decades younger than I whose locks flow down their backs, who have not a thread of gray. Last night, when I put on my fur hat, one of my students said I looked "imperial."

Two years ago, Mike Riz disappeared, and in the spirit of capitalism, no one at his salon would tell me where he went. The eighteen months it took to find him were a trial, but when I found him at his own eponymous salon, our reunion was sweet.

"Ah! Honor!" he said, and he gave me a big hug and then his card and cell phone number so we would never again be parted. Like John Sahag, he is Lebanese, and just yesterday, as he worked, hair dryer in one hand, brush in another, he rehearsed the answers to questions for his citizenship exam: What is the separation of powers? Who is the governor of New York? He never knew Congress had two houses! As he blew me dry, he said again how he had missed my hair all those months we were separated, and then he did what he always does at the surprising moment when my hair is all dry: he lifts and pulls it away from my head, twisting the brush this way and that, lifting and brushing so that it falls back in waves, then with his hands massaging my scalp upward, the hair again falling and settling. Every time he blows my hair dry, he does this. And every time he does it, we laugh. "Beautiful," he says. "Beautiful."

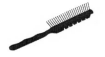

# My Wild Hair

MARIA HINOJOSA

**M**y brother and I thought we had made a major hair-dressing discovery. He was eight and I was six, and we were trying to find a way to make our somewhat unruly hair look more like our friends Bobby's and Lisa's, nice and flat and straight.

We had discovered that if you cut off the top portion of our mother's stocking, it became a tool to silkiness. We would pull the thigh of the stocking over our heads, down to just above the eyebrows, and tie the top part like the end of a sausage. If we put the stocking on after a bath and slept that way, the next morning we'd have smooth hair, and though it looked a little awkward, we knew early on that with flat hair, all would be good in the world that day.

My new country didn't understand my home country's hair. I was a mixture, a mestiza of Mexican, Caribbean, Spanish, Indigenous, and African (still no DNA proof, but this is my best guess). So my hair was unruly. Curly. Frizzy. Loud.

My birth country was Mexico. My new city was Chicago. In both I had problem hair.

It was all about keeping it down and flat. I was in such deep agony about the perpetual frizz that I begged my mom to take me to get my hair ironed, and I meant with an actual iron. She didn't think much of the idea. She said no and even called me *una loquita*—a little crazy girl.

In junior high school, something called Hair So New changed my life. I sprayed on the conditioner and suddenly the tangles were gone. That meant I didn't have to wear my nylon stocking cap anymore. The next hair development was feminism. At the height of the movement in the 1970s, short hair became hipper. That helped a lot, since my hair never seemed to grown straight down anyway—why not keep it short? In high school, a few years later, curly perms were all the rage, so I cut all my hair off and had a hip little 'fro till my senior year, when I let it and my armpit hair grow out.

At Barnard College, in New York City, I began to accept my "not the norm" looks and my Latina identity. I stopped cutting my hair, and soon after, watching the movie *Eu te amo*, I found my new hair role model. Her name was Sonia

Braga. Back then, her long black hair was curly, unruly, and wild. I knew I could never be her, but I could try to make my hair look like hers. And that hair was almost half of the mystique around Dama Braga.

As I came to accept and even love my wild hair, it became a way for me to feel power that I had never experienced. Physically, I am limited. I am only five feet tall. But with my full hair out and a pair of five-inch platform shoes, I had presence and I gave off the air of being tall. I saw that once I accepted my hair, I could accept myself in a deeper way. And soon I really did have the Braga hair—and then the fun started. I remember nights when I danced and swung my head and my long, luscious curls, dancing myself into a delirium. My wild hair was an essential part of feeling free, uncontrolled, and in the moment.

> *As I came to accept and even love my wild hair, it became a way for me to feel power that I had never experienced.*

I have happy hair memories of my first foray into television as a journalist on a local New York PBS station, in the early 1990s. It was a group of us talking around a table, and no one paid much attention to my long, curly hair. But soon after, when I was asked to anchor my own show, I was told to tie my hair back and make its distinctiveness disappear. I think they wanted me to be a Latina Talbots model. It was not all that becoming, but it taught me an important lesson: being on TV meant I would have to conform to someone else's idea of how I should look.

When CNN called in 1996, asking me to join them as a correspondent, one of the first items I put in my contract was that they could not dictate my hairstyle. And they agreed. But as I got older and the on-air look became more competitive and conformist, with big, glossy hair the new normal, I learned to blow out my hair, and then it became a habit.

*But soon after, when I was asked to anchor my own show, I was told to tie my hair back and make its distinctiveness disappear. I think they wanted me to be a Latina Talbots model.*

Now that I run my own media company, I decide how I want to look on camera. And I always struggle with my hair and my look. Always. Only on rare occasions does it look just right. I have become accustomed to getting out of bed and praying to the "hair gods" that when I unclip it, the hair will fall perfectly into place. I learned the clipping technique from a Dominican hairdresser, who showed me that it was a way to keep the body and curl. Most every night I roll my hair into two loops on top of my head with special bobby pins.

But nothing anyone could say about my hair affected me

as much as what my artist-husband said in the middle of a heated argument over how much time I spend working. Everything about me had changed because of work. "Even your hair is corporate now!" he charged. "It's short and straight, like everyone else's!"

I was horrified and wounded. My husband looked at my hair now and saw corporate, put together, and uptight—the opposite of Sonia Braga!

I made a promise to myself to prove my love to my husband by letting my hair grow out as long as I could. I would become the wild woman again, to honor him and prove my love through my hair. I had the best of intentions, but in truth I also wanted to see if, after fifty, my hair would still cooperate and grow. I took on my hairdresser too, who is a hard-core believer in the school of Over Fifty Women Should Never Have Long Hair. And for three months, I was going to stop coloring it too.

I also checked my calendar for upcoming TV shoots, to make sure that I could get away with not being on camera during that period. But the entire challenge came back to one thing: love and my husband, whose own gorgeous hair made me fall in love with him.

When I first met him in 1988, German had a Dominican 'fro. We connected instantly, but we were both in other relationships. Two years later, I ran into him at the Village Gate, at their weekly Salsa Meets Jazz concert. My hair was in full Sonia Braga mode, and I danced in Braga style. His hair had grown and he was sporting a long, curly ponytail. The sight of this masculine, muscular man with a ponytail made me feel weak at the knees. I knew that night I had found the one. And I knew his new hairstyle had something to do with it.

After hours of dancing, I asked German up to my apartment for tea. Instead of jumping on me like a dog, as we got comfy on the sofa he put his gorgeous head of hair on my chest and just lay there. My first act of loving touch with my future husband was to stroke his hair and run my fingers through his ponytail, while I marveled at the tightness of each curl and the butter softness of each lock. Our hair sealed our relationship, and it is still at the heart of it.

What do I mean? The greatest act of love I can show German is to comb out his hair and braid it. I brush it back in long swipes and then weave it into a power braid, usually with a Native American leather tie. When he is painting a canvas, his hair can go wild, one half black, the other half white, with strands of hair everywhere. But mostly he prefers to wear it pulled back and tight. Forceful. Controlled. No loose ends.

During big fights, we have been known to throw hair into the ring. "I swear," my husband said once, "I will cut off my hair! Just like you did before you gave birth to our son. Cut off all your hair without even telling me!"

I've learned that hair in arguments is always a dangerous thing. And so are promises. So I didn't tell my husband about my plan to grow out my hair as a guerrilla-tactic response to his critique of my so-called corporate hair. At the end of October, I stopped cutting and coloring it and started wearing it curly. A gray streak came out over the right side of my head. I was shocked by how quickly the gray took over. My young staffers told me the streak made me look kick-ass and powerful. I hated it because it reminded me that I am over fifty. My staff noticed, but my husband didn't for quite some time. Hair grows slowly, and he's an artist and in his own world, not focusing on me the way my colleagues do at the office.

The truth is that the promise to honor my husband was also a promise to honor my younger self. I am hopeful that a woman who wears her hair long and wild like Sonia Braga is saying something about feminine beauty. She is saying that it is imperfect, unpredictable, and that the wild-hair thing is a thing of beauty, not a look to be shunned and blow-dried away. After years of keeping my hair in order both in length and in color, I wanted to show that wild women exist behind masks of perfect hair.

Since the promise, I haven't cut my hair (except to trim it slightly to get it to grow more) for six months. I haven't had hair this long in eighteen years. I haven't worn it curly so many days in a row in over a decade. And I love it. I feel younger and, yes, sexier. Where has German been during all this time? I think that because the change in my hair was so gradual, he got used to the new me little by little, without any fanfare.

As I WRITE this I am traveling back from a week in my parents' home in Mexico City, where I went to purposely disconnect. I left their home only twice. I was content just to bask in the shadow of the Iztaccíhuatl and Popocatépetl volanoes. And during all those days, I never once tied up and clipped my hair. I let it be as wild, long, and curly as it is.

And yes, I do this for love. Because I love myself more like this and because this way I show my husband my love, not in words or deeds, but in hair.

As soon as I got home from Mexico, German saw what had been before his eyes for months. He told me that he loved my hair. I smiled and said I was glad he noticed but I didn't tell him why I had done it.

That weekend, late one night when the moonlight came in through our Harlem apartment window, I stood next to a candle I had lit and saw the shadows of my long, curly, loud hair. I called German to the bedroom and said, "This wild head of hair is in honor of you, *mi amor*. This is the real me. The real Sonia Braga in me. And I love you for inspiring me to bring her, and me, back to you."

# Love at Last

· · · · · · · · · · · · · · · · · · · · · · · · · · · · · · · · · · · · · · · · · · · · · · · · ·

## JANE GREEN

The first time I fell head over heels in love with a hairstyle, I was at university, sitting in a darkened movie theater, mesmerized. I wanted to be Kelly McGillis in *Top Gun*. I wanted her flight jacket, I wanted her man, but most of all I wanted her blond, curly bob.

My hair was not altogether dissimilar to hers. More frizz than curl, and a natural auburn, it hung down to my waist. Surely if I cut it, dyed it, scrunched it dry with lots of mousse, I could miraculously turn myself into Kelly McGillis.

Patience has never been a virtue of mine, nor comfort in my skin, particularly when young. At eighteen, at university in Wales, away from my London home for the first time, I would have done anything to turn myself into someone else. I had no idea, back then, that who I was was enough. All I knew was that I didn't belong, I didn't feel good enough. I was too tall, too big, and too ungainly and had a halo of thick curls that I wished were straight. Perhaps if I emulated a Hollywood star, perhaps if I changed the one thing it was so very easy to change, I might, finally, fit in.

A friend and I found the one late-night drugstore in town and giggled our way round the aisles until we found a home highlighting kit and a pair of scissors. Back in our hall of residence, I gathered my hair in my fist and hacked it off into an uneven bob. The lack of symmetry didn't matter, I told myself: my hair was thick enough to hide a multitude of sins. My friend spent the next three hours pulling thin strands of hair through a myriad of tiny holes dotted all over a plastic cap sealed tightly around my head. We smeared bleach everywhere, and all the while I dreamed of my glamorous new life with a blond bob. But the reveal proved the bleach was no match for my natural auburn. My hair was now an orangey shade of yellow, or perhaps a yellowy shade of orange. More Big Bird than Kelly McGillis. Disaster though it was, this was just the beginning of my hair-transforming experiments.

I was born with a mop of thick, curly hair. It was the kind of hair that elicited compliments from strangers in the winding streets around our home in Hampstead Village.

It formed a halo around my head and flowed halfway down my back. Hairdressers went into raptures of amazement. And I would have done anything to change it to a sheath of shiny silk.

I was raised in a family where looks counted. My mother is tiny and beautiful. My father has an eye, an appreciation, for good looks. While clearly loved, I often felt like the invisible child, hidden away, buried in books, longing for a happiness I could only read about.

Back in the seventies, formal photo shoots were the order of the day. As children, my brother and I would be sent off to photography studios in the quiet suburbs, my hair pulled and blown out by my fastidious mother into a sleek hairstyle that even now I remember adoring. This elegant girl was who I wanted to be all the time; this was who I was in my mind.

Straight, glossy hair was beautiful. Rampant, frizzy curls were not. At school, the popular girls had the hair I coveted. Silky and blond meant popularity, likability, success. My curls were creative and shy; they never quite fitted in. But I could lose myself in books, in other, easier worlds, and convince myself that if I cut my hair and dyed it blond, the romantic hero could fall in love with me too.

Everything in high school was about my looks, the crowning glory being my hair, the tumble of curls moussed into submission, the front blown out to a sleekish wave. I would happily forgo makeup but never went anywhere without my professional-grade hair dryer with the all-important nozzle. After graduating from high school, I went InterRailing, traveling around Europe with one backpack and a sweaty train ticket in hand.

*I wanted so badly to be someone I wasn't, wanted so badly to find a way to be comfortable in my skin. Hair was simply the easiest thing to change.*

My travel companion brought a professional backpack with combined sleeping bag that weighed more than she did and was almost as tall. Like Cheryl Strayed in *Wild*, she had to crouch down on the floor every day to hoist it onto her shoulders. Free spirit that I was, I chose instead to bring a tiny backpack, the type of backpack my kids now sport every day to school. It contained T-shirts, shorts, underwear, and a huge professional hair dryer with accompanying brushes. As long as my hair was perfect, I had a chance at feeling good enough.

That fateful night at university, the first night of my experimentation with hair, I was genuinely stunned to discover I didn't look like Kelly McGillis when I was done. I looked like me, with bright yellow, shorter hair. A couple of years later, obsessed with Holly Golightly, I took a pair of scissors to my bangs and was again shocked I didn't look like Audrey Hepburn either.

I wanted so badly to be someone I wasn't, wanted so badly to find a way to be comfortable in my skin. Hair was simply the easiest thing to change, the most obvious aspect of my appearance to alter.

At twenty-one, I learned how to straighten my hair with a round hairbrush and the all-important professional hair dryer with the narrow nozzle, tame those wild curls into something resembling sophistication, resembling *good enough*. Products came and products went, and my hair stayed straight for years.

At twenty-eight, I left my job as a journalist to write a novel. Within three months there was a bidding war for my first book, which went straight onto the best-seller lists. I was overwhelmed by an immediate best seller, fearful of the attention, fearful perhaps of being *seen*. I had more attention than I had ever had before and was desperately trying to navigate a life that suddenly seemed to be in the public eye. I had fame of a kind, success, and, for the first time in years, financial stability; the only thing missing in my life was a boyfriend. I somehow convinced myself that making a drastic change to my hair would bring about drastic change to my life, and so I did. My new haircut was too short, much too short, a boyish, butch haircut that didn't suit me. I had left the hairdresser in tears. But change did indeed occur. I soon met the man who would become my first husband, and finally, after all those years of hoping to be loved, I stopped trying to change myself. I had finally found someone who loved me, who didn't care if my dress size went up or down, and who certainly didn't care what my hair was like.

Our wedding day saw me going back to Audrey Hepburn for inspiration, this time without the short bangs. I had an elaborate "updo," my curls first straightened, then elaborately twisted into a tight bun on the top of my head. Looking back at the photographs, I see the melancholy in my eyes. I looked like I was trying to be someone I was not, marrying a man I knew, deep down, was not the right one for me. I didn't consider my own feelings, whether I loved him, whether I thought we were a good match. The fact of his loving me was—and how sad I am to admit this—enough.

*I scraped my hair back in a ponytail, eschewed makeup, and took the kids to the beach every day, where we made picnics and built sand castles.*

I was a very good wife, despite the constant feeling that I was in the wrong place, had made the wrong choice. As if in an arranged marriage that I had arranged myself, I would make this work, would accept that I had chosen with my head rather than my heart. I suppressed the nagging suspicion that we would not grow old together and stepped into the role of the perfect wife, throwing all my energies into keeping a good house, cooking, entertaining, and always looking perfect.

I grew my hair long but changed the color. Initially dark, once my twins, my third and fourth children, were born, I went straight to the hairdresser's and became blond. Long became short, became the classic bob length. I blew my hair out every day, was coiffed and immaculate, the very picture of a trophy wife, all of it hiding the turmoil I felt inside, knowing I was living the wrong life, with the wrong man.

For most of our marriage, I was the sole breadwinner, supporting our entire family writing my novels, but I didn't want to be. In my affluent Connecticut town, trying to fit in, I wanted to be the Stepford wife, wanted to pretend to be the housewife, married to the successful husband, lunching with the girls.

We separated after seven years. The seven-year itch. Those words would play in my head over and over leading up to our seven-year anniversary. I knew it would be a turning point, that we couldn't continue pretending to be right for each other, pretending to be happy. When we split up, it felt liberating to dye my hair straight back to its natural auburn brown and grow it long. I moved into a tiny beach cottage, lived in shorts and T-shirts, for the first time in my life not using the outside to try to present an image to people of who I wanted them to think I was.

I scraped my hair back in a ponytail, eschewed makeup, and took the kids to the beach every day, where we made picnics and built sand castles.

My landlord was around a lot that summer, in a nearby house. Slowly, over shared coffees and glasses of wine and against everyone's better judgment, for I was so newly out of my marriage, we fell in love. I remember walking out the front door to get the mail as he happened to be passing. I was still in my pajamas, makeup-free, my hair tousled and messy. He says now that he fell in love with me at that moment, when he saw who I really was.

Later he confessed he didn't like my makeup and high heels,

or my blown-out, perfect hair: "helmet head," he called it. He liked me entirely natural, my hair curly, caught back in a beach-messy ponytail, in flip-flops and T-shirts, with nothing to hide behind.

During that summer, falling in love with the man I would later marry, I learned to stop trying to be someone else. I learned that I didn't need to hide behind an image, that even if I was just me, someone wonderful would still love me, think I was perfect, no matter what I looked like.

My hair is now streaked with gray, and, recently, blond. It is long; sometimes straight, sometimes naturally curly, depending on my mood. I'm still unnaturally attached to my hair dryer, but on the days I don't have time, I am finally safe in the knowledge that after all these years, whatever my hair is like, I am lovable, and loved.

# The Cutoff

. . . . . . . . . . . . . . . . . . . . . . . . . . . . . . . . . . . . . . . . . . . . . . . . .

### DEBORAH FELDMAN

Until I was eight years old, I wore my hair in two braids, a hairstyle my grandmother retained from her Old World past. My peers sported pageboy bobs, and I desperately wanted short hair as well, as my braids were often made fun of, but I could not conceive of how to go about persuading my grandmother to let me get my hair cut the way I wanted. She was a Holocaust survivor who had experienced agony and grief that I found frightening and unimaginable; because of that, I could not figure out how to justify this one demand. However miserable my unconventional hair made me, it could not even begin to register on the scale with which she measured suffering.

In second grade, I hit upon a clever scheme. I came home from school one day with an urgent message from the lice inspector. She was fed up with my long hair, I reported. It had become too difficult to examine. I could not return to school until my hair was trimmed to a manageable level. The inspector had said no such thing; she had simply flipped through my head of hair, layer by layer, before finally pronouncing me clean, which hadn't always been the case. But the little harrumph she emitted when she undid my braids and saw how much hair I had was just enough to get me thinking: Could I pass off her minor frustration as something more?

In the 1990s, lice were rampant in all the schools in Williamsburg, especially the religious private school I attended, which was run by the Satmar rabbinate and housed thousands of students in close quarters. I had had my share of lice. Those dangerous chemical treatments had not yet been outlawed; I often went to bed with my head lathered in a purple shampoo, the smell of which was so all-powerful it took away my olfactory abilities for weeks, but the morning after, my white pillowcase would be covered in heaps of brown specks, some still quivering. There was the special comb too, with very fine, long teeth that my grandmother used afterward, trying to get at any eggs left behind, from which a whole new crop of lice could hatch. I had such thick hair, and it made my eyes sting and water to have that comb scraped through every strand for what felt like hours.

My grandmother had lived with body lice in the concentration camps; to her these banal head lice were "bubkes"—they hardly presented a threat. She combed away matter-of-factly, humming a tune, and indeed, her work was so thorough I never suffered from a repeat infestation.

My grandmother's head had been shaved twice, once in Auschwitz, and once again after she married my grandfather, a member of the Satmar Hasidic sect. When I told her my hair would have to go, off it went. It seemed she wasn't as attached to those braids as I thought she might be. We went to the little salon located on the slanting side street that overlooked the Brooklyn-Queens Expressway, which was run by two bodacious Hispanic women. One of them pulled my virgin hair too tight on a round brush, and when I cringed, she consoled me with this lingering maxim: "Mama, you gotta suffer for beauty!" I would ponder that phrase for years to come.

I was besotted with my new hair when I gazed into the mirror two hours later, admiring its clean lines. My shiny, straight hair seemed perfect for a pageboy style. I was so happy to go to school the next day, to finally experience the blessed relief that came with looking like everyone else.

It's true that the haircut did not fool my peers into thinking I was *just like them*. After all, nothing could erase the shame of my parents' divorce, not in the Satmar community, where the integrity of the family unit was paramount. But I remember that my new hair lessened some of the acute pain and self-consciousness I had been saddled with until then, and surely I was teased less often, once I no longer had lumpy braids for others to point at and mock.

The Satmar Hasidic community is one that places tremendous emphasis on uniform appearances; it is understood that there is only one way for agents of God to dress, and even if you look perfectly modest, it is felt that difference, in itself, is a form of immodesty. Failure to blend in is probably the most egregious social crime one can commit. That's why I kept my hair in that same style for more than a decade, in the hope that by dint of my conformist appearance, I would gain the acceptance I craved. Now I attribute much of that longing to the common adolescent urge to fit in; teenagers can be so harsh, even Hasidic ones, and my survival instincts kicked in to protect me from the worst of their venom. I experimented in occasional minute variations in the thickness or the length of my bangs, the barest hint of layers, but always there was that square china-doll shape that framed my face the way it did every other Hasidic girl's in my neighborhood. Eventually, I would join the married women in my family by shaving my hair and donning a wig instead, as required by strictly enforced tradition.

The day I got married, a stylist came to the house a few hours before the wedding and teased my hair over my tiara, inserting the teeth of a white tulle veil in the stiffly sprayed mound. The next morning, since I was now a new bride, my aunt took out the electric razor I had been gifted as a part of my bridal trousseau, plugged it into the bathroom wall, and ran it over my scalp in swift, assured movements. Clumps of stiff, dark hair fell into the sink, and I remembered that moment so long ago at the hairdresser's, when my soft, golden strands had floated to the floor of the salon. I had been so happy that day to let go of that weight.

Yes, I was relieved now also. There was a complex mixture of emotions brewing within me then, and I didn't allow them to surface, but I now remember quite clearly that relief was a disproportionately large ingredient. There was that familiar joy of finally being the same, of being initiated into the community as a full and legitimate member, which my new headgear would proclaim to all those in doubt. Until my marriage, I had never been fully accepted. Despite my china-doll haircut, the lingering effects of the scandal of my parents' divorce had always rendered me something of an outcast, but now that I was in a marriage of my own,

*The next morning, since I was now a new bride, my aunt took out the electric razor I had been gifted as a part of my bridal trousseau, plugged it into the bathroom wall, and ran it over my scalp in swift, assured movements.*

with another member of the community, I might hope to cancel out the shame of where I came from.

And yet, my shaved head did not buy me full acceptance

either, although it purchased a kind of tolerance that, for a while, seemed like it would be enough. People seemed more inclined to forgive my ignominious origins, my inferior family connections. I felt not so much an outcast as low caste: it was the bare minimum of membership.

A year later, I stopped shaving my head during pregnancy, although I still had to keep my head covered. There was no one to inspect me. I was free from the monthly ritual of showing up at the local *mikvah* to be pronounced kosher and ready for procreation. My hair grew in black now, because no light reached my head, always tucked underneath a turban or a wig.

*Eventually I threw away my wigs. I abandoned the community that had forced me to wear them.*

In my seventh month of pregnancy, I went to a salon in New York City with two inches' growth and asked them to shape it. The hairdresser spoke to me in a pained whisper. She thought I was a cancer survivor. She could barely contain her tears at the idea of a pregnant cancer survivor. It was too complicated to explain the truth to her, and besides, she gave me a big discount.

My hair grew in slowly. For a while it was lackluster and thin. Then I started taking off my wig on hot summer days, when I was secretly attending classes at Sarah Lawrence, and slowly it came to life. My head could breathe again. My hair lengthened and lightened, but most importantly, it lifted itself off my head. No longer matted and compressed under a burdensome weight, it blew about in the breeze, relishing its newfound freedom. I hadn't realized how much I missed that feeling. Putting the wig back on became something I dreaded. As I covered my head each time I prepared to return to my community, I felt as if I was stifling much more than my scalp. It was as if my very thoughts were shrinking.

Eventually I threw away my wigs. I abandoned the community that had forced me to wear them. Ever since my son had been born, I had felt my desperation to leave increase exponentially as he grew older, learning to speak Yiddish instead of English, having his hair cut into side curls; and before he was enrolled in yeshiva at age three and officially outside the realm of my influence, I fled. We started our life over in New York, where he learned to speak English in three weeks.

Each time I went out in public with my hair uncovered, I felt more real, more solid. As it grew, inch by inch, I felt my realness increase, and could feel my footing in this new, unregulated world stabilize.

Five years after I left, a friend of mine reached over and tucked a long lock of hair behind my ear, telling me, "You know, I just realized, you're one of those women who hides behind her hair."

"What do you mean?" I asked.

"I've never seen you wear your hair up. It's as if you use all that hair to hide your face, or your self."

I was surprised at her comment. I had never thought of myself as someone who hid from anything.

I have a lot of hair now. I have cut it only a handful of times since first growing it out. It has seen many summers; its strands are various shades of golden. I brush it carefully each morning and put conditioner on the ends; when I go out into the world, it feels like a lion's mane. The last stylist who blow-dried my hair ran her fingers through it when she finished and said, "Honey, you have power hair."

It's true. Like the shoulder pads of the eighties, or the pantsuit of the nineties, my hair gives me character and individuality. I do not so much hide behind it as arm myself with it.

Still, my friend insisted. "You shouldn't hide your face. It's beautiful. You would look very good in a twist or a bun." She gathered my hair in her hands and lifted it off my neck, as if to see. "There! Now I can see those cheekbones."

I glanced at my reflection in the mirror behind us, but I did not see what she saw. I saw instead the broad, eastern European cheekbones of my grandmother, whom I had never seen with her hair. In the Satmar community, married women's hair was viewed as a sinful and dangerous tool of temptation. Now, cutting it, or putting it up, felt like a concession. I was like Samson. My hair was my strength. I would never again allow that strength to be undermined.

Recently I tried to drag my eight-year-old son to the barbershop to get his hair cut. Like my own hair, his grows so quickly; it's shiny and thick, the same burnished golden color of those clumps on the salon floor so many years ago. He cried and refused to get in the chair.

*My hair was my strength. I would never again allow that strength to be undermined.*

"What's the matter? Don't you want to get all that hair out of your eyes?" I asked, looking at his thick mop with concern. It seemed in danger of turning into a mullet.

"No. I like it long," he insisted, brushing the hair aside.

I looked at him in surprise, realizing suddenly that this was his way of asserting his individuality, and that unlike me, he didn't have to resort to subterfuge to wear his hair the way he wanted to. I smiled.

"OK," I said. "You grow it as long as you want."

# Glory

· · · · · · · · · · · · · · · · · · · · · · · · · · · · · · · · · · · · · · · · · · · · · · ·

RU FREEMAN

**A** few days ago, all these many years into my adulthood, I
posted this on Facebook

> Haircut. I.e., morning during which I writhe in agony wondering if
> I even need a haircut, wanting a change, resisting a change, picking
> out a different hairstyle, printing out those different hairstyles, and
> then working myself up into such a state that I plonk on the chair
> and state emphatically that I LOVE MY LONG HAIR, and coming away
> after paying a ton of money for a nice chat, shampoo, and ½ an
> inch off the ends. What is wrong with me, people? What is WRONG
> with me?

to a chorus of commiserating murmurs. I went for the said haircut and returned to upload a photograph that shows me largely
unchanged, albeit slightly buffed.

My obsession with hair is partly cultural (Sri Lankan culture values thick, long hair) and partly personal (the emphasis people placed on my hair as I grew into my teenage years). We inherited great hair genes, my brothers and I, with dark, sweeping locks that seem not to age. My oldest brother grows his down to his waist and when pressured to cut it by our mother, when she was still alive, would invoke Samson. My other older brother, a die-hard Socialist, who sets aside large parts of his salary to help strangers and friends, sees no contrary tendency in purchasing expensive product for his hair.

When I was a very young child, there was never a fuss made about my hair. As a kid, I was marched off to the barber along with the boys, and once, I famously received sideburns because the barber could not distinguish my skinny-boy body from that of my brothers and assumed I was a third son. But once I turned thirteen and my mother decided it was time for me to *begin to look like a girl,* people outside the house started to express admiration for my hair.

*My oldest brother grows his down to his waist and when pressured to cut it by our mother, when she was still alive, would invoke Samson.*

Whether it was because the quality of it was somehow, miraculously, exceptional in a country whose women almost invariably had long hair, or because I did not have much else in the way of notable female assets, it was my hair that people spoke about. Within the extended family, my paternal grandmother, who was never very fond of me (an antipathy carried over from her feelings about my mother), would sometimes stroke my head and bemoan the fact that my hair was not good enough. No curls, she'd say, dejectedly, pronouncing it "kay-rels," the part I latched onto so I could make a joke of a comment that stung. But she was the exception. At school, in the days before things turned sour between us (and by then I would have learned, in my wicked, adaptive way, to take pride in the fact that their envy was still intact), my classmates would cajole me to audition for the new advertisements that were being broadcast on TV, for a shampoo we'd never heard of, Sunsilk. (TV itself had just arrived in Sri Lanka, gifted by the Japanese along with Japanese television sets.) Other friends begged to spend recess, which we called intervals, undoing my ponytails and braids and running their fingers repeatedly through the hair that seemed to weigh more than my head. The nuns at the convent I attended—those reliable killjoys—insisted on tight braids that hid the beauty of our hair, but I took pleasure in ripping out the rubber bands and practicing a bouncy swagger that swung my waist-length ponytail from side to side as I walked. It stood to reason then that I was soon expelled from that school and left without a backward glance.

From the convent I was moved to a fancy private girls' school, where I was admitted not on my own merit but on account of my mother's fame as a renowned teacher of English literature. It was a school established by the more insidious Christian missionaries who were smart enough to cloak their God-given right to spread goodwill among us Buddhists in laissez-faire derring-do. These girls laughed at the slogan by which I had been ruled at the Holy Family Convent: "Simplicity is the keynote of a Familian." Here, there was no prescribed length for our uniforms, and hair could be managed any way we pleased. It was not an easy transition. These were young girls with notions of fashion and a lot of money. Hair dryers were the norm. I didn't possess one (my family did not possess many electrical gadgets, not even a radio). I improvised with a single table fan that had been placed in my bedroom, as the only girl in the family, a title I bore with great pride. To dry my hair, I pulled out long sections and held them in front of the fan until the mass of it fell straight down my back. I hadn't know it then, because I didn't grow into it until I was an adult, but I had what was an amalgamation of my mother's and father's hair. When wet and left to dry, it displayed the "kay-rels" of my now deceased grandmother's heart, and when combed out it fell in waves that, within a day, would turn straight. I didn't need hairstyles because my hair styled itself.

Fast-forward to the year of our Lord 2005. I was rooming with another writer, Nina McConigley, at the Bread Loaf Writers' Conference, and I saw her holding a smallish object

I had never seen being used before. Like most Sri Lankans, I don't wash my hair every day, almost never blow-dry it, and use only oils for styling and those, rarely and sparingly.

"What is that?"

"A flatiron."

"What does it do?"

"It straightens your hair," she said, and then she proceeded to demonstrate on a few strands of my hair.

What smooth sleekness! What miracles! Here was a chance to augment the versatility of my hair. I could, I figured, wash it and let it be curly on one day, wavy the next, straight the third, and a sheet of glass the fourth! Nina gave me tips on purchasing one of these contraptions, and indeed, when I returned home, I bought one. I hardly used it over the next years, while I eked out my existence, I thought, *on the sidelines of history*, writing articles and stories and eventually a book. The flatiron came into its own only this past year during a second book tour, and only because I had been shown—while being primped for my author photograph—the use of an electric curler. A curler, it seemed, could work on my untamable hair only if I first flat-ironed parts of it. And though my preference is still to let my hair just be, I confess that I've played with this a few times, enough to feel I had some skills I could hand off.

Not long ago, I was visiting Anjali Singh, a senior fiction editor on the New York literary circuit. Anjali was the one who had, years ago, encouraged me to drop the 487-page novel I was shopping around and complete the one I had just begun. That encouragement had lead to the publication of my first novel, *A Disobedient Girl*. Surely I should have remembered what I owed her when I sat down to read a book to her older daughter. The woman in the book we read was using plastic curlers. Anjali's daughter didn't know what they were, and I explained, conjuring up an image of high fashion as she listened with rapt attention. Oh, I could just feel the yearning in her little-girl body, a yearning that took me back to my own girlhood. Anjali, forgive me, I couldn't resist.

"But," I told her, "nowadays there are electric curlers, you just roll up your hair"—and I rolled up mine to show her—"and when you take it out, you have pretty curls."

She nestled up to me with adoration in her eyes. "Do you own one?" she asked.

"Uh-huh," I said, "and your mom, if you ask her, she'll probably be able to get one for you."

YES, AS A kid I had not only drunk but wholeheartedly believed in the Kool-Aid my mother fed me, referring repeatedly to hair as "a woman's crowning glory." The biggest lie I ever told my mother revolved around my hair: I claimed that there was a free styling offered by the hairdresser when I needed to go to a very important party at the age of fifteen. My mother's biggest outrage at my oldest brother came when he accompanied me to that same hairstylist (for his own hair) and encouraged me to ask for a Farrah Fawcett number that decimated both the highly prized length and quantity of my hair. And the one time I ran away from home was because, after I had been suspended from the convent (the nuns could get creative with their punishments, the more guilt-inducing the better), my mother swore that all my misbehavior stemmed from my obsession with my *bloody hair*! Then she marched off to fetch a pair of scissors so she could hack it off. I remember sitting on the floor under my table as she had instructed me, wondering how long it might take her to find a pair of scissors in our chaotic house, where nothing was where it was supposed to be and where most rudimentary tools simply did not exist, and realizing that there was nothing for it but to flee. And so I did, running barefoot through the streets of Colombo, taking my precious hair with me.

It wasn't hard to believe in the drama of hair, given that my grandmother, my mother, and her sisters all had beautiful manes that grazed the backs of their knees. Indeed, family lore has it that my grandmother was once forced by the nuns at her school to cut off some of her hair. Apparently, her hair pooled on the floor as she sat up in a tree, cast in the role of Asokamala, the female lead in the most famous love story of Sri Lankan history, interfering with the progress of the prince tasked with wooing her from her perch. My mother's combing

and braiding of her own hair was mesmerizing to behold, as
was the way her plait moved against her hips as she walked.
I was not yet a woman, but I swore I'd acquire whatever
glory was being handed out through this mane with which
I had been blessed. As I grew up, I learned to organize my
clothing around my hair: what-
ever looked best with whatever
my hair happened to be doing
was what I wore. It never failed
to work its magic. At least on the
surface, I could manage to look
like I was sailing through times
that tested my spirit: finding and
losing boyfriends, surviving two
schools where I was ostracized
by my entire class for long periods, leaving my island home to
come to northern Maine for col-
lege, defending my undergraduate honors thesis, jobs that
spanned thirteen states, marriage, motherhood, graduate
classes to which I went with an infant in a Snugli, unemploy-
ment, and all the way to walking alone into black-tie galas in
New York City. So long as I had my looping, falling tresses,
I could convince myself that I was not simply passable but
utterly magnificent, that I could turn any moment around
in my favor.

> *As I grew up, I learned to organize my clothing around my hair: whatever looked best with whatever my hair happened to be doing was what I wore. It never failed to work its magic.*

It was those words spoken by my mother about the importance of my hair that made it feel like the most natural thing
in the world for me to spend most of my student-job wages on
Pantene shampoo and conditioner, while my fellow internation-
als on our snow-filled campus in Maine purchased bottles of
Suave for ninety-nine cents.

"How could you spend so much on shampoo?!" a student
from Nepal asked me the first time we were driven to Kmart
to acquire supplies.

"Because it's my hair!" I said, fully expecting this to suffice
as explanation and dismissal.

This hair was not just my hair; it was my badge of courage,
my shield, my vice, my tiara, and my salvation all rolled into
one. In the summer of 2002, I made a series of decisions that
left me living once more in Maine with no job and no money to
call my own. I had given up work that I loved and had moved
with the intention to write, but this was practically impossible
while going through the ups and downs of pregnancies and
childbirth and the unforeseeable difficulties of raising three
very young children among, as I liked to point out regularly to
my Caucasian husband, *all these white people!* I was a good
and devoted, if somewhat eccentric, mother, but motherhood
had never been a holy grail for me. And so, despite the in-
comparable gift of my children, I felt only the weight of being
useless in the world, given all I had expected to do during this
phase of my life.

"I have nothing to give," I mused one day, sitting at the dining table while three small people sat before their afternoon snacks and regarded my sad face. I was wrapping my hair around my fingers as I said this, and in the silence that follows such utterances made in the presence of children who can neither understand nor help, it came to me that I did have one thing I could give: my hair. I had not cut my hair short since I was thirteen years old. All my haircuts were mere trims. All my haircuts since would remain trims. But for a glorious afternoon in the midst of such despair, I felt wealthy. This hair that had always been my gilding, I could and I would cut it off and do something useful with it, something that had nothing to do with personal vanity, although it surely had something to do with a certain vanity of the spirit that seeks to impress itself in some way upon the world. My husband approached the task with the enthusiasm he brings to kitchen renovation projects. I doubt he understood the enormity of the moment, but he participated fully in getting it done precisely and according to the instructions provided by Locks of Love. Bands at the top and the bottom, and a clip that took off much more than a foot of hair. Once mailed, the hair would be made into a wig for a young girl or woman who had lost her hair during chemotherapy.

Of course the aftermath was predictable. I went to the hairdresser to get it styled into something other than the jagged mess I now had, and came back with a beehive. (The only woman of color in the entire magazine of haircuts I was shown at the salon wore a beehive, so I guess the stylist assumed it would suit me too.) I said nothing but came home sobbing. I tried to rinse it out and then to pull it down from its high perch, to no avail. I tied a scarf around it and went about looking like a Russian peasant for a few days. And then I decided that this was no way to behave in front of three impressionable girls. It's just hair, I told myself, it'll grow. And though it hurt like hell to have my oldest daughter say, as I climbed into her bunk bed to kiss her good night, "You don't look like my mother," indeed it did grow.

Most of the time the things we do shape our children more than our words ever could. Following the advice of my mother, who was channeling her own ancestors, I made sure to shave the heads of each of my three daughters before they turned one, the ritual most likely to guarantee the development of gorgeous hair. "You have to do it before they speak their first word," my mother told me. "Otherwise the shock of it will delay their speech." There they sat, each in her turn, one minute like every other floppy five-month-old, the next their features sharply in focus beneath their shining, tender, naked heads. I am not convinced that the inability to articulate their feelings about the change meant they weren't horrified. To this day, they behave as I do in the lead-up to and the aftermath of a haircut, displaying in exact sequence intense self-evaluation, courage, excitement, pleasure, and dismay over the most trivial of changes.

I listen sympathetically. I murmur soothing words. I know I'm raising girls who will grow into women who will carry around a talisman with the power to morph, when needed, into weapon or cloak, wrap or jeweled ornament, comfort or strength. I can see them walking through life nursing private anxieties but exuding a certain joie de vivre, their heartstrings linked invisibly to each strand of their beautiful hair. The older ones buy their clothes, as I usually do, on consignment, on eBay, or at end-of-season sales, and the youngest simply inherits. But from the age of nine, each of them has visited real hairdressers. I can't afford Mason Pearson boar-bristle hairbrushes, but the ones I buy them are the best I can find for what I *can* afford. The two swimmers and runners have argan oil and shampoo that protects against chlorine and sun damage. The one with the fine blond locks gets hair treatments.

When I take them home to Sri Lanka, my father, in the sadness of my mother's absence, sometimes sits them down and rubs large quantities of coconut oil into their heads as they wrinkle their noses. I disregard their baleful glares. I smile, remembering such moments in my own childhood. Yes, I cursed and swore (silently, of course), but I knew that those hands held powerful intention. Sometimes here, in my American life, I massage wishes into my daughter's lives, holding each lush and unique mass, each fistful of dark and light hair in my palms, rubbing potions into one, rinsing foam off another, braiding and twisting, ceaselessly caressing not their heads but their innermost selves. I do these things, and I see them growing up, leaving me, having babies. I see them shaving heads, brushing hair, rubbing oils. I see them as goddesses passing on this same, easeful message of self-love.

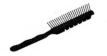

# Act Tresses:
# Hair as Performance Art

ELIZABETH SEARLE

### Jackie Kennedy and Audrey Hepburn

My family moved a lot. I was the perpetual new girl: a skinny late bloomer with buckteeth decked with metal braces. I found refuge in elaborate pretend games I played with my sister till I was well into my teens, and in old movies we watched with Mom. I was fascinated by Audrey Hepburn in *Two for the Road*—the way she transformed from the "ugly duckling" of her schoolgirl group into a radiant young wife and later a jaded, glamorous jet-setter.

You can change yourself through your looks and styles, I was starting to see. We grew up with a framed photo of JFK above our dining room table. Years before I was born, Mom saw JFK speak as a presidential candidate, his famously fab hair tousled in the wind. He looked, Mom reported reverently, "like a Greek god."

Would JFK have risen to power and immortality if he'd had more ordinary hair? In the biblical Samson story, hair *is* power. Who can calculate how much those heads of lavish Irish hair helped the Kennedy brothers? Not to mention Jackie. Her hair.

Another fascination I shared with my mom. Jackie Kennedy with her preternaturally wide-set eyes, dramatic dark brows, deeply dazed regal manner, and darkly intelligent stare and the shiny helmet of hair she wore into battle beside her dashing husband.

*Years before I was born, Mom saw JFK speak as a presidential candidate, his famously fab hair tousled in the wind. He looked, Mom reported reverently, "like a Greek god."*

As Ted Kennedy memorably said of Jackie in his eulogy: No one looked like her or acted like her or sounded like her. Or, Teddy didn't need to add, had hair like hers.

I knew I'd never have hair like Jackie's. But I dared to hope for Audrey Hepburn hair when I first saw *Roman Holiday*, one of my mother's favorite films. How dramatic is the haircut scene and Audrey's transformation from princess to gamine whose bouncy short-cut hair reminded me of Mom's. And what I hoped my own straighter, oilier hair might somehow someday become. If I "took care of it." As a kid, that meant Mom giving my sister and me what we dubbed "sha-baths," a combo of shower and bath. We'd sit in the tub under the full shower stream and Mom on her knees would scrub our hair, hard. Green Herbal Essences shampoo bubbled over my long hair and bare back. A lush green-foamed, sweet-scented princess cape. Not that the preteen me was any princess. Not on the outside.

## I Dream of Jeannie

My first hairdo of choice, when I was five, was a princessy ponytail. I had to flip over so Mom could grasp all my long brown hair and twist it, hard. Mom was a science teacher who kept a dissected cat in a plastic bag in our garage; she was no wimp. Her hands were strong. With no-nonsense force, Mom would pull my hair up. It had to be high like a crown, like the harem hairdo on *I Dream of Jeannie.*

Deftly, Mom would snap my ponytail into place with a double-twist motion and a single "ponytail maker"—a number 8–shaped rubbery band decked with twin plastic marble-size balls in different groovy colors. The then "shocking" pink was my fave.

When Barbara Eden in *I Dream of Jeannie* nodded her head hard to cast her spells, her blond ponytail bobbed and gleamed as if magic itself. Even my plainer ponytail bounced like a real pony's tail. It was worth all the hard brushing and twisting needed to create ponytailed perfection. I was learning this lesson young: beauty hurts.

My mom had been pictured on the cover of a science magazine when she was in her twenties: a dazzlingly glamorous lab technician intently concentrating on her test tube, her pursed lips so darkly lipsticked that they look, in the luminous black-and-white shot, black. Her brown hair too looks lushly black—like Elizabeth Taylor's hair. I loved the fact that my mother had been on the cover of a real magazine, like a movie star. Though Mom denies it, I always believed she named me partly after Elizabeth Taylor, considered for decades to be the most beautiful woman in the world.

*It was worth all the hard brushing and twisting needed to create ponytailed perfection. I was learning this lesson young: beauty hurts.*

Mom, a dark-haired beauty and pioneering career girl in the 1950s, had been dubbed by her Philadelphia roommate First Most Beautiful Woman in the World. Mom worked then in a lab, testing soaps and beauty products. She knew the dark arts of conjuring beauty. As I grew up, Mom regularly used Loving Care to touch up her dark hair. The chemical smell and pasty brown substance seemed anything but loving and left blood-dark stains on her head scarves. But

I loved the results: Mom "magically" maintaining the richly brown hair color I'd inherited. I was happy to be my mother's hair heir. But I couldn't picture being happy in my mother's quiet life now that she was no longer a big-city scientist but a high school biology teacher and housewife.

### Gloria Steinem and Ali MacGraw

Gloria Steinem was my own teen-hood icon, one I'd fixated on myself, not via my mom. I loved Steinem's aviator-style wire-rimmed glasses and her long, straight, center-parted hair, streaked with ashy blond, simple yet striking.

I wore glasses too. I entered seventh grade wearing ill-chosen dark plastic stop-sign-shaped frames that prompted my South Carolina school's mean girls to crow: "She look like a dog in them glasses." I vowed to myself that someday I'd escape to snowy collegeland, like Ali MacGraw did in *Love Story*— another of my mother's favorite films, one she didn't let me watch when I was little "because it's too sad."

But to gawky me, the film offered a glimpse of a better to-morrow. The tale of a smart girl who escapes to Radcliffe felt hopeful even though she dies before her senior year. I loved to imagine a world ruled by brainy chicks like Ali, smartly at-tired in her black tights and black-framed glasses, crowned by her simple yet sexy "do." Center-parted, shoulder-length, dark brown hair. Like . . . mine! Only it looked way better on her.

My senior year, my family's cross-country moves landed us

in Arizona. In my fourth high school, I nabbed the lead in the school play and published stories in the Chaparral High literary magazine, my long brown hair streaked now with blond highlights by the fierce Phoenix sun, my pallor and acne tanned away. Plus, I was old enough for contact lenses. So I wasn't Ali MacGraw, but things were looking up.

### "Can I Touch Your Hair?"

How important *is* hair in life? How big a role did my own auburn-brown college-girl hair play in initially captivating my future (and present) husband? A turning point came as I sat at age nineteen beside my future mate, then a worldly twenty-eight, in his bachelor apartment on what I later learned he called the make-out couch.

"Can I touch your hair?" John, who had a major head of hair himself, asked me.

John came from a family of major hair. His mother had what she dubbed "many-colored hair," which no doubt caught his dad's eye on the same Oberlin College campus where I met John. By then I knew that, like plumage on birds, bright hair attracts mates.

My mother and father had fallen in love at first sight, dancing to "Love Me Tender." They married a mere four months later. But my mom had been twenty-nine at the time, after almost a decade on her own, having her "career girl" adventures in Philadelphia. I married at the tender age of twenty-two, some of my own adventure seeking still untapped.

Together, John and I left the cradle of our midwestern college town to head east—where I found myself wanting bigger hair to match my bigger ambitions.

## The Kate Bush Perm and
## The Accidental Aniston Cut

It seemed like a good idea at the time. The first perm: in my midtwenties when I was still in graduate school and we could barely afford groceries, much less pricey salons. But I loved the rocker Kate Bush's wild mane of lioness hair.

This was back in my own wildish days. I was trying out experimental fiction at Brown University's MFA Program, while experimenting with my hair too. Years of perming wound up frying my once-shiny hair into a too-bushy frizz, a do that matched the stressed-out frenzy of my postgraduate aspiring-writer years, scrambling for literary success in Boston. Not that there weren't some swell parties along the way in the nineties when my first books were published.

My husband describes women like guitars: "acoustic" and "electric." I may have started as an acoustic girl, with loosely curled hairdos and natural-looking makeup. But by the mid-nineties, I was trending toward electric, with darker lipsticks and shorter skirts and higher heels. My teaching job at Emerson College planted me in posh downtown Boston, where I had my hair more expertly permed.

Then motherhood hit. Nothing was the same after our son was born, including my hair. Like most new moms, I barely had time to brush, much less style. I also hadn't had time to follow the swinging-singles show *Friends*. But when I emerged from my baby-besotted daze long enough to get a haircut, I wound up accidentally Aniston'd, my wavy hair woken up and amped up by angled layers. My hair was nowhere near a Jennifer Aniston level of lushness and sheen, yet her signature layers gave middle-aged me—sidelined from the writing life—a lift. Inside, as well as out.

### Best Performance by a Ponytail

The segue from writing fiction to writing librettos for an opera and a rock opera in my forties marked another era change for my hair. This time, the hairstyle I eventually chose was not like anybody else's. It was my own and my hairdresser's concoction, designed to fit the new me. As a writer of literary fiction and a college teacher, not to mention a frazzled mom, I'd kept my hair and clothes simple.

But around the time my lively son was old enough to stop running me ragged, my writing career took a dramatic turn. At an age when many writerly careers are on the wane, I reinvented myself, stumbling into a project that brought my work national attention for the first time, and even a touch of notoriety.

For years I'd been obsessed with the infamous 1994 Tonya Harding/Nancy Kerrigan Olympic skating scandal, in which the skater Kerrigan was whacked in the knee by an assailant and suspicions focused on her rival skater Harding. I'd first written about Tonya and Nancy in a novella, *Celebrities in Disgrace.* But when I hit on the idea of turning their larger-than-life tale into an opera in 2005, I found my work drawing a new level of attention. I wound up writing the librettos for both an opera and a rock opera and talking for years, several times on national TV, about the shows and the lurid knee-attack scandal itself.

*When I emerged from my baby-besotted daze long enough to get a haircut, I wound up accidentally Aniston'd, my wavy hair woken up and amped up by angled layers.*

I also found myself drawn into a world I'd always loved from afar: theater.

So it was that on a spring night in 2006 in my midforties I found myself driving from a Harvard Square theater rehearsal of *Tonya & Nancy: The Opera* to a nearby mall on an urgent mission to purchase a clip-on ponytail.

The lovely singer playing Nancy Kerrigan in our opera had all she needed to embody Nancy and belt out her "Why Me?" aria—except the long ponytail. Incredibly, photographers from the AP were coming to capture our girls in costume, amid our strange and heady surge of media attention.

Normally a cautious driver, I sped down Route 3 to the Burlington Mall, ran in just before closing time, beelined to a garish booth. Breathlessly, I tried on several high-end ponytails. I splurged on a glossy seventy-dollar model. Triumphant, I raced to my car with my ponytail still clipped on, more gleeful than the sullen teens I galloped past.

What have I been doing with my life? I found myself thinking giddily in my car, glimpsing myself in my rearview mirror. My Aniston cut had grown too long, but the clip-on ponytail revitalized it. I roared back to the theater, greeted like a hero for having found the perfect ponytail.

What a thrill—like playing dress-up dolls, only better—to watch as our perfectly attired and ponytailed Nancy and Tonya emerged that night to a barrage of AP flashbulbs. Somehow buying that ponytail marked a turning point for me: it made me realize that theater writing was more than a passing fling. And that I needed a new look for my theatrical writing life.

## Big Hair

My mommy-hair days came to an abrupt end the day ESPN Hollywood called. When ESPN said they were sending a cameraman to my home in two hours for an interview about the opera, I hung up in a giddy panic, wondering if I should tidy my living room or do my hair. It was a no-brainer. I seized a ratty brush from my nightstand and bent over to give my hair a vigorous brushing. The aging brush snapped in half.

I phoned my usual salon, could not get in, and then dialed a trendy new place I'd noticed. The stylist told me my plentiful yet baby-fine hair would "respond to product." Loading my hair with foam, powder, and spray, she teased it so hard my scalp ached. But when she was done, my hair had magically expanded. I looked less like a middle-aged mom and more like a wild and crazy librettist who'd cooked up an Olympic-scandal opera.

Over the subsequent busy years of interviews and rehearsals and further, crazier adventures writing a rock opera, my big-hair style helped me muster some extra moxie. I was getting my professional mojo back. I began giving livelier fiction readings too. With my hair high, at age forty-eight, I won a Literary Death Match medal.

Unlike a perm, teasing is temporary. So I can switch from casual carpooling-mom hair to big hair as needed. My do is a tad retro. But it works for me. Better than beta-blockers or Botox, having my hair curled and teased lets fiftyish me feel a little onstage oomph.

"Hair, makeup, wardrobe," a long-ago TV ad mused. "Where would an actress be without them?" Or an actress at heart, like me? All my life, I have taken on different personae with different hairdos. My mother is the opposite. After cutting her long hair to begin her working life in her early twenties, Mom has basically stuck with the same short, bouncy haircut and the same Loving Care hair color, on into her eighties.

She will never be ready, she's decided, to go gray. But she was up for a relatively late-in-life career change. In her fifties, she shifted from teaching science to earning a new degree and taking a new job as a children's librarian. Another quiet profession, but one in which she could act out her own love of theater by reading aloud to kids, energetically voicing the different roles. Yet "Mrs. Searle" always looked reassuringly the same to her young students—as she does to me, still, when I visit her in sunny Arizona. She moves less briskly now, but she has the same level, blue-eyed gaze and same game, lipsticked smile. Mom, with her Jackie O. sunglasses and her short Audrey Hepburn hair, always the same warm shade of brown. I'm the one who's changing my hair color as I age, opting for lighter highlights to soften my face.

I see now that for me, hair has always been a performance art. In the newest version of my *Tonya & Nancy: The Rock Opera* script, still evolving after two professional productions, I added a line awarding Nancy Kerrigan "Best performance by a ponytail." Even for those of us living far from the Olympic-size world stage, our hair is a kind of performance we give throughout our lives.

### "I Like It Different"

Nowadays, in my early fifties, I am happily schizo with my hair: keeping "acoustic" in my day-to-day housekeeping and teaching life, with my shoulder-length hair hanging loose, but changing things up to my more "electric" style when I need to be "on."

"Everything comes and goes," Joni Mitchell sings, "marked by lovers and styles of clothes." And, I'd add, by styles of hair too.

Hillary Clinton, famous for her shifting hairstyles, has said wryly that over the years she has grown not only older and wiser but "blonder." Like Hillary, I have found mixing in golden-brown streaks to mask the scattered white in my still-brown hair helps brighten my midlife look and outlook, like Christmas lights in midwinter.

Everything does indeed come and go. Styles change as quickly these days as the ever-shifting celebrities who set off one hair craze after another, while rising and falling with Internet-powered speed themselves.

Still, we each primp hopefully for our own little star-turns. My mother at age eighty-four still treats her hair with Loving Care. New hairstyles give me a boost when life gets a bit blah, whether from the pressures of motherhood or middle-aged angst, or worries over what lies beyond. Luckily, I have little time lately to fret over my advancing age.

Mixing it up with youthful high-energy theater folk is one way to stay young at heart. Recently in New York City, in the spring of 2013, I slipped into the ladies' room of a music studio where our rock opera was being performed as a staged reading showcase. The ladies' room was still redolent with the heavy-duty hairspray of the actresses, some of them Broadway pros. I pulled out my own purse-size bottle of hairspray, breathing deeply to calm my nerves. And I felt, as I inhaled their spray with mine, a sense of sisterhood with these starlets.

Like them, in my own smaller way, I primped as if I were suiting up in battle armor. A few well-aimed spritzes of spray made my hair, and my spirits, rise. Head and hair high, I opened the door to face my audience.

# Remembering Sandra Dee

## HALLIE EPHRON

It's 1958 and I'm ten years old, a skinny kid, all elbows and knees, a long face with big eyes under furry caterpillar eyebrows, sitting on a stack of telephone books in the chair at Mr. Latour's Beauty Salon, where my mother gets her hair done once a week. I've come here often with her, but this is the first time Mr. Latour is cutting my hair.

Everything in the salon is pink or gray, including Mr. Latour, who has thick gray curls that remind me of a French poodle. He's washed and cut and brushed my mother's short hair until it's a glistening tour de force, a virtual Christmas wreath of curls neatly encircling her head.

Now it's my turn.

I sit in the chair, my feet dangling off the ground, and stare at myself in the mirror. My hair is thick, jet black, and more or less straight. My mother appraises me with a sour look. She tells Mr. Latour that if he doesn't fix my hair, soon I'll start looking like Veronica Lake.

I don't know who Veronica Lake is, but I know from my mother's expression that this would not be a good thing.

*Everything in the salon is pink or gray, including Mr. Latour, who has thick gray curls that remind me of a French poodle.*

Later I learn that Lake is a sultry movie star, memorable more for the way she wore her silken tresses covering one eye than for her talent. Sultry isn't yet in my wheelhouse.

"Can you cut it like this?" I ask. I show Mr. Latour a picture of June Allyson that I've cut from a magazine. She's a fresh-faced blond with short, curly bangs and a perfect pageboy.

Mr. Latour makes a show of examining the picture. Then me. I squirm under his gaze. He and my mother trade smirks.

He wraps my neck with a strip of scratchy crepe paper, then snaps open a cloth and drapes it over me. Turns the chair so I can no longer see myself in the mirror. Then he picks up a shiny pair of scissors. The scissors feel cold against the side of my face. *Snick.* I shiver at the sound.

*Snick. Snick.* With each sound, chunks of hair fall to the ground. When he stops, the speckled linoleum floor is covered with my hair. He makes a few last snips, then removes the cloth and the crepe paper and whisks errant hairs from the back of my neck. He turns the chair so I can see myself.

"Voilà," he says.

June Allyson is not staring back at me. I've got bangs that look as if they've been chopped off with a paper cutter. The sides look hacked off too, and though one side obediently curls under, the other side flips up, giving me the dreaded Bozo the Clown look. I feel like I'm going to be sick.

"Much better," my mother says in a chirpy voice as she applies fresh lipstick and fishes her car keys from her pocketbook.

It's a good thing no one asks me what I think, because if I try to say anything I'll burst into tears. All the way home I'm thinking, I hate my hair, I hate my hair, I hate my hair.

At home that night, I try to salvage the mess. Slowly, methodically, I take one strand of hair after another, wrap it around my finger, and anchor the curl in place with crisscrossed bobby pins. In the morning, I brush it out, trying to coax it smooth and turned under. Before I leave, in the mirror I catch the faintest glimmer of June Allyson.

I walk to school, holding my head high and steady so my hair won't get mussed. I imagine that I'm a model gliding down the runway. If I have to turn, it's point, pivot, turn. If I have to lean over, I bend at the knees.

By that afternoon, I've forgotten about being a model, along with my glamorous pageboy. As usual, after school I wheedle my way into a boys' softball game. As usual they stick me way out in right field.

The sun is shining, it's hot, and as I wait for the ball to come my way, I notice that my socks have scrunched down into my Mary Janes. The backs of my ankles are coated with dust from the playground's asphalt. I can see from my shadow that my pageboy has erupted on one side. I run my fingers through it, again and again, trying to coax it back under. Inevitably, it's at that moment that a fly ball with my name on it sails past.

A few years later, I bring Mr. Latour a picture of Sandra Dee. She's another wholesome, bright-eyed blond who stars in *Gidget*, the quintessential Malibu movie about a girl who gets herself a surfboard, shoulders her way into an all-boy surfer gang, earns their respect, and (of course) falls in love.

Sandra Dee's hair is a shorter version of June Allyson's, pumped full of air. There's a fancy French word for it: *bouffant*. But we call it the bubble.

By now I realize that Mr. Latour is more or less a one-trick pony, so I'm not surprised when I get the same haircut he always gives me. But I leave feeling optimistic because the movie magazine ran not only a picture of Sandra Dee's hair but also a detailed diagram with instructions for how to replicate it.

Pin curls won't do it. I've saved up my allowance and gotten myself a set of rollers at J. J. Newberry. Each inch-thick wire cylinder is stuffed with a prickly brush. Before going to bed, I set my hair, wrapping a strand of hair around each roller and running it through with a plastic anchor. A hairnet holds the rollers in place. Thus armored, somehow I manage to sleep. The only part of this that feels good is when I release those sausage curls the next morning and give my scalp a good scratch.

The trick to the bubble is teasing. *Tormenting* would be more apt, since this involves back-combing until all the hair on my head is

*It's a good thing no one asks me what I think, because if I try to say anything I'll burst into tears. All the way home I'm thinking, I hate my hair, I hate my hair, I hate my hair.*

standing up in tangles. Then it has to be smoothed and patted and shaped into one massive hair ball. Waves of hair spray turn the spun confection rigid.

My mother, who never has to set her hair and whose hair always looks exactly the same, barely looks up from her newspaper when I come down to breakfast with my new do. I realize that as long as my hair isn't hanging in my eyes, she's not going to notice.

A few months later, I modify the look after seeing *Last Year at Marienbad*, a French art film in which I believe nothing happens except Delphine Seyrig swans about in black and white, looking utterly fabulous with her pale skin and her black hair smoothed back in a sleek bouffant with a single curl tucked artfully around her ear.

It's that curl that captures my imagination. It's called a *guiche*—French for "spit curl." While Ms. Seyrig may have used spit to keep hers in place, I use clear nail polish to glue mine to the side of my face.

I wear a bouffant with a *guiche* the same year I win an enormous plaque proclaiming me Sixth-Grade Girl Athlete of the Year. Sixth Grade's *Only* Girl Athlete is more accurate, because by now the boys won't let me into their pickup games and I've stopped asking. There's just one girl in my class who doesn't think it's weird that I still play ball after school on the playground. Sometimes she plays with me, but more often it's just me standing alone on the basketball court, working my way around the key.

With the ball balanced on my palm, I center myself and take aim, imagining the clean arc the ball will take before it whooshes through the hoop. And sometimes that's what happens. But I'm doomed if a stiff breeze kicks up and disturbs the hair mats that I lacquered that morning. It takes two hands to hold down my hair.

It never occurs to me that my obsession with my hair might be diminishing my athletic potential, so it's just as well that in seventh grade I give up sports completely. I also refuse to go back to Mr. Latour. Instead I tag along with my older sister and get my hair cut where she does. I keep trying to explain to hairdressers how I want them to cut my hair.

In the sixties, I want *That Girl* Marlo Thomas's flip. (Big surprise, my hair will only flip on one side.) In the seventies, it's the figure skater Dorothy Hamill's swingy wedge. (My hair is too thick to swing.) A few years later, I want Farrah Fawcett's feathered do. (Turns out I don't have the patience for the amount of daily blow-drying that this requires.)

I achieve a modest success in the eighties when, trying to look like Jennifer Beals in *Flashdance*, I get a perm. I actually look a little bit like her character, Alex, whose spectacular break dancing earns her a scholarship to a dance conservatory. That year I even dress like her too, cutting the necks out of all my T-shirts and sweatshirts and wearing my sneakers with slouchy socks.

It's not until years later, around the time that my daughter starts obsessing over her hair (pouffy bangs, high ponytail in a colorful scrunchy), that I stop investing energy in mine. It starts to go gray and I let it. Now it's more salt than pepper, and I'm fine with that. I keep it short and uncomplicated. After a shampoo, I towel it dry, give it a tousle, and I'm good to go. There are no celebrity snapshots I can bring to my hairdresser to show how I want to look because there's not a single American movie star who looks even remotely like me.

Still, some things don't change. The hair on one side still refuses to turn under. My hairdresser, who's never heard of Bozo the Clown, says it's a cowlick and I should learn to love it. It's

my hair's personality asserting itself, and after all these years
it's not about to change.

When my daughter balks at going to my hairdresser—in
tears, she tells me he makes her look like a monkey, and I
know better than to say I think her hair looks cute—I tell
her about Mr. Latour, who did a perfect job on my mother's
hair and a perfectly awful job on mine. I tell her she doesn't
have to go back to my hairdresser, ever, and I trot out old
pictures of myself to show her the lengths to which I used to
go to get my hair to behave.

My daughter is a terrific athlete. Sweeper on her soccer
team. She anchored the 4×4 relay in track. She can even
pole-vault. When I suggest she might have gotten her athletic
ability from me, she does a double take.

I tell her about my Best Girl Athlete award and she gapes
at a picture of me taken that year. I try to explain about
Sandra Dee and Delphine Seyrig. She's unimpressed.

She tells me that the term for hair like mine in that picture is *choucroute*. While this lacks the elegance of *bouffant*
or *guiche*, I have to admit she's right. I do look as if I've got a
perfect mound of sauerkraut on my head.

"So what teams were you on?" she asks.

I explain that when I was her age, there were no sports for
girls. No soccer. No track. All we had were physical educa-
tion classes where we spent most of the time lining up by

height and taking turns catching and throwing a ball. It was boys-only on the ball fields.

But still, I tell her that in elementary school I tried to be a player. A little baseball. A little basketball. And who knows, I might have gotten really good if I hadn't been so obsessed with my hair.

# Maids of the Mist

KATIE HAFNER

On the credenza in my office stands a framed black-and-white photograph, taken in the early 1960s during a family outing to Niagara Falls. We are aboard the *Maid of the Mist*, wearing heavy rubber raincoats with sturdy hoods. My aunt, uncle, and cousin, who had come with us, look stoic, even thrilled to be drenched by the mist thrown off by the powerful falls. My father must have been the photographer, because he isn't in the picture. My sister and I, ages six and four respectively, appear vaguely unhappy, no doubt holding out for the promise of hot chocolate at the end of the ordeal. But it's the look on my mother's face that makes an indelible impression: Head bowed, she is gripping her hood at its base, wrapping it tightly around her slender neck. She does not look happy to be there.

For the many years I have owned this photograph, I've assumed she just didn't like the cold, wet setting. It wasn't until recently, studying the picture anew, that I entertained the idea that there might be another reason for her dark mood: *the effect Niagara Falls was having on her hair.*

Bodies, and everything attached to them, have long dominated the fine minds of the women in our family, some of whom were prominent scientists and accomplished musicians. My own limitations in the physical sphere were clear to me when I was very young. At age eight, I was held up for scrutiny by my grandmother, who voiced her doubts about whether my figure would ever amount to anything.

My mother and sister were especially incandescent in their beauty. By the time she was fourteen, my sister had blossomed into a younger version of my mother—a rare combination of sinews where sinews mattered, an Audrey Hepburn neck, and perfect bone structure. My mother was gifted in both physics and mathematics, and for men of a certain type, the beauty-brilliance combination was an attraction like no other.

As for me, I came to hate my body, especially my nose, which in the course of my own pubescent bloom had tripled in size. It was a replica of my father's nose, directly proportional in size to his. I was so frightened of myself as a child that I once asked a close friend of my mother's whether I was pretty. I was sure she would give me the benefit of the doubt. Instead, she was honest: "You're pretty enough," she said curtly, only to go on at rapturous length about my sister's physical gifts.

But I possessed one thing my mother and sister did not: naturally straight chestnut hair. And both of them envied me for it. Theirs were heads covered with thick and unruly frizz, the curse of many a Jewish woman who wished she didn't look quite so Jewish. Indeed, women mess with their hair because it's the easiest thing to change, the ultimate accessory. Many say their hair sends a message to the world about who they are. When it came to the women in my family, they wanted to send a message to the world about who they wished they weren't. More precisely, they wished their Jewish looks weren't so indelibly etched on their heads.

Of course, many women want another woman's hair. If yours is curly, you wish it were straight. If it's black, you want it blond. If it's blond, you want it to look more ethnic. If it's thick, you think it's too bushy and would prefer it "fine," even wispy. I always had the feeling that my mother and sister could not for a minute fathom the fact that such a silken mane had been wasted on me. And wasted it was. My own genetic good fortune was lost on me. I took little comfort in the fact that my hair required no maintenance, that all I had to do was wash it with whatever shampoo I found in the shower and let it hang dry. When I was very young, of course, their envy barely registered, but even as I grew older, I took little comfort in knowing that my mother and sister admired my hair.

In fact, my hair was the object of envy among many of the females in my life. Not long after that trip to Niagara Falls, my mother left my father, and my sister and I eventually came to live with him, our stepmother, two stepbrothers, and a stepsister. My sister and stepsister, close in age and at constant war over boys, detested each other. But they hated their hair even more than they hated each other. Throughout their teenage years, the girls spent thousands of hours and no small fraction of their weekly allowance forcing straightness upon their naturally kinky hair. In the late 1960s and early 1970s, long before the advent of flatirons, Frizz Be Gone, keratin treatments, and a portable blow-dryer in every bathroom, they subjected themselves to endless attempts at getting their hair to look like mine.

My sister went so far as to lay her locks straight down on the ironing board, using a clothes iron to flatten it. After an unfortunate singeing incident, the effects of which wafted through the house for hours, she abandoned the clothes iron and stuck to setting her hair in large pink plastic hair curlers, then sitting for hours wearing a plastic bonnet hair dryer. My stepsister used empty frozen orange juice cans. After washing her hair, she would pull it up on top of her head in a ponytail (using, yes, a rubber band). She would split the ponytail into a half-dozen or so sections, then wrap each section around a can, which she would then attach using extra-long bobby pins.

Rain is the nemesis of women with frizzy hair. My stepsister's ritual for walking home from school in the rain was to part her hair down the middle in the back and wrap each side section around her head, turban-style, clipping it flat against her head with bobby pins, then donning a rain hat.

Although I was vaguely aware of how miserable all of this made the females with whom I lived, the fact that I was side-lined—a mere observer to their hair mania—made *me* miserable. I felt left out. I lived in my sister's shadow and remained in awe of her nose of appropriate proportions, her large breasts, and her tiny waist. Frizzy hair was just part of the package. I begged and beseeched: Please put curlers in my hair too. They ignored me. So I made one or two of my own ham-fisted attempts at rolling my hair. The result was a neither-here-nor-there effect—vague curls that lasted a few hours, then reverted to strands as straight as I beams.

The only consolation I took in my hair was that it provided evidence that I was not, as a neighbor had once observed, a "Xerox" of my father. I adored my father but did not want to look like him. What separated me from him was my hair. His was wavy. Mine was straight. With the flawed logic that kids often employ when trying to square themselves with the world, I decided that our different hair meant we didn't *really* look alike.

Then one day I took a close look at a photograph of him at age twelve or so. There was the signature nose, the thin lips, and the receding chin. And his hair was as straight as, well, mine. I panicked and asked him about it. Oh, yes, he said, his hair was naturally straight, but shortly after that photograph was taken, one night at summer camp a gang of bullies shaved his head while he slept. When it grew back, *it was curly.* This evidence of a one-to-one genetic transfer sealed it. I was forever doomed.

As I grew older, I still failed to appreciate my mane. And in the way that comments from childhood can trail after us for decades, the "pretty enough" judgment tossed off by our family friend had taken root in my psyche. "Pretty enough" became my self-identity, and there wasn't much I could do about it—with one exception. When I got to college, I decided that if one key to my mother's and sister's beauty was their God-given hair, then that was something about myself I could change. So I got a perm. If frizz is what I wanted, frizz is what I got. I looked like a cartoon of someone who had just inserted her finger into an electrical socket, but I couldn't have been more pleased. I sent a photograph to my mother. "Why would you want to look any more ethnic than you already do?" was her response.

In my twenties, my fixation on appearance melted away as I entered an overly smug and earnest phase of life. I was wrapped up now in being a young radical in the mold of Jane Fonda, whose own lovely locks seldom went unattended, mind you—just take a look at her acceptance speech for the *Coming Home* Oscar. I found I had no patience for my sister's continued preoccupation with hair. "Look at the sheen on that girl's hair!" she said once while we sat in a restaurant. I followed her gaze and saw a woman with a head of long, straight, very shiny dark brown hair. Sheen? Really? I chastised my sister for caring so much about something so superficial. I told her she had been captured by classic Marxian false consciousness. At that moment, I thought less of her for caring more about the sheen of someone's hair than about the Trilateral Commission, or the daily fascism found on the *Wall Street Journal*'s op-ed page, or whatever capitalist conspiracy I had decided to rail against that week.

In my thirties, my political fervor mellowed into a liberal latte lover's complacency, and I grew interested once again in looks. But now I transferred my concern to my daughter, Zoë, whom I had with my second husband (had I had children with my very Semitic-looking first husband, my mother once remarked, "the child would have looked like E.T."). Zoë was blessed with looks not from my side but from her father's, a handsome collection of Irish and French blonds and redheads with a dash of Cherokee mixed in. My own hair, still full and dark and very straight, ceased to matter much to me. For I was inordinately proud—secretly, of course—of her hair. I had feared she would be one of those newborns born bald or with a head of hair so light it was undetectable. But my daughter emerged with ample amounts of light brown hair, which soon turned very blond; then, by the time she was five, it was thick to boot. Still better, both my mother and sister pronounced Zoë generally "stunning."

My sister died suddenly and far too early, at the age of fifty-five. It would be easy to say that the enormity of her death made all the fuss over looks and hair seem silly. But for me, at least, all that fussing took on an importance that, while my sister was alive, I hadn't been able to fully appreciate. Her preoccupation with her hair became important to me because it had been so important to her. Now, four years after her death, when I conjure an image of my sister at the end of her life, the first thing to appear in my mind's eye is her hair, still long—and kept meticulously straight.

*Now, four years after her death, when I conjure an image of my sister at the end of her life, the first thing to appear in my mind's eye is her hair, still long—and kept meticulously straight.*

At around the same time my sister died, my mother began fretting less about her hair and more about growing old. Well into her seventies she kept it long and pulled it back into a loose bun high on her head. Now she wears it short, so short that it's nearly impossible to detect any curl at all. The thousands of hours she invested in it, now moot, will never be regained.

As for me, my own thick, straight hair is now a perk of the past. When I look in the mirror, I hope those are gray roots I'm spotting but know they are patches of skin, follicles gone fallow. My thinning hair has turned into not just one problem we see shampoo advertised for, but *every* problem we see shampoo advertised for: it is dull, lifeless, damaged, *and* brittle, with random strands of frizz thrown into the sorry mix.

My daughter, now twenty-two, seems perfectly relaxed with her hair. She does nothing but wash it, condition it, and let it hang dry. In other words, she doesn't obsess. She just takes good care of it and brushes it with the same Mason Pearson "Detangler" she has used since she was small. It's gorgeous. And you should see the sheen.

# Hair in Three Parts

. . . . . . . . . . . . . . . . . . . . . . . . . . . . . . . . . . . . . . . . . . . . . . . . . . .

## DEBORAH JIANG-STEIN

**1.**

One day when I was around twelve, I tiptoed into my parents'
bedroom when no one was home and snooped in their dresser.
What I discovered spun my world out of control. Buried in the
top drawer under silky slips and perfumed bars of round soap,
I found a typed letter my mother had written to the family at-
torney, and in just one paragraph I learned I had been born in
a prison in West Virginia, to a chronic heroin addict.

Prison? Who's born in prison? I dove into emotional lock-
down, the news so traumatic, and that day a wedge divided me
from my parents—because I never told them I'd learned about
my roots. My mother had already told me a few years earlier

that I was adopted, and the world knew too—this caramel-colored, racially ambiguous girl in an all-white family.

No one knew why I'd shut down, not my family, not my teachers, no one. I didn't even know. I'd locked myself up in my own prison inside, where time and memory blurred. I was afraid of the world, terrified of people. Most of all, I was scared of myself and hated myself: I'm the daughter of an inmate. I'm bad, I thought, bad because I was born in a prison.

But in my day-to-day life, I was the daughter of two academics, two English professors, my adoptive family, who were as confused as I about what locked me up. In fact, I kept my birthplace a secret until I was an adult in my twenties and told a friend. At the same time, curiosity drove me to learn more. I just couldn't metabolize how a baby can be born in prison. After some investigating and detective work about my background, I learned that my birth mother and I lived a year together in the prison until authorities removed me from her cell. She was just beginning her ten-year sentence.

Prison is no place for a baby, the warden eventually decided, so I began the journey to foster care and, later, adoption—which sounds now like a fairy-tale ending to a tragic beginning.

But by the time I was eighteen and estranged from my parents, law enforcement in Seattle, where I had grown up, was hunting me down for petty crimes, mostly drug-related, in three states from California to Washington.

Twenty years after I found the letter, I met my birth family through a search agency and was devastated to find out that my birth mother had died. But they gave me a treasure, the photo album she'd kept in prison and forever after. It was all she had left of me. Beneath the sheen of a three-inch ragged-edge square of cellophane affixed inside her photo album, a single thread winds around the center of a few strands of my baby hair. On other pages, filled with my baby pictures, her love bleeds from the cracked corners of the black construction paper.

These are the few treasures I've inherited from her, along with two tiny knit sweaters and a yarn toy, and a blood-carried disease she possibly passed on to me—all pieces of a fractured story that have helped fill in the blanks of what I learned in the letter.

## 2.

Rome, Italy. My father took my brother, my mother, and me on his sabbatical year so that he could finish one of his books on John Milton's *Paradise Lost* or some other epic poem he studied. I was in third grade, eight years old.

One day, my mother was sick, maybe with a flu, I can't remember, but she was too sick to braid my hair the way I always liked to wear it for school. My father's big, clumsy fingers, thick as the smuggled Cuban cigars he smoked, braided my hair, a mass of black hair like a troll doll, into weak twists.

*My father's big, clumsy fingers, thick as the smuggled Cuban cigars he smoked, braided my hair, a mass of black hair like a troll doll, into weak twists.*

On my run to the bus, the bands in my braids snapped out—the only time I could remember my hair flying free. By the time I took my seat on the bus, shame washed over me.

I'm exposed, naked, I thought, frantic about this undressing.

I wanted the power and boldness of Medusa to save me from the humiliation. We'd just studied the legend in Greek mythology, at the Overseas School I attended in Rome. Medusa's hair transformed into serpents—this is how I imagined I looked without my braids. But I didn't have her boldness, not on the inside. I was terrified of people, and the fear turned me mute at times. Most of all I was still scared of myself.

One day a decade later, back in Seattle, where I lived on my own after graduating from high school, I was in the hair salon for a cut. My stylist, Johnny—one of the slick, fast-talking thugs I hung around with who also smoked weed in the alley behind the salon between his customer appointments—said, "You have a few bald spots in back. You know this, right?"

When I thrust my fingers into my thick, wavy, shoulder-length hair, Johnny took my wrist and guided my hand to the back of my head. The shock of these spots, the size of a quarter, and smooth and hairless as my cheek, horrified me. I yanked my hand away.

At first, I thought it was damage from all the hair product. I loved my hair. I took good care of it. No more braids. I let it fall to my shoulders, free and wavy, and sometimes humidity thickened it. I was a loyal hair product consumer, with mostly gel and spray, and an easy believer in all the promotions that corporations bombard us with in advertising.

But no, Johnny said, the baldness wasn't a side effect of hair products. He said it was alopecia areata, spot baldness caused by stress.

I'm damaged, I thought, and in an instant felt uglier than I already did. I'd grown up in a white family, a multiracial girl in the 1960s, at time when civil rights and race blending were just coming into public view. On top of that, I didn't know what races I was, only that my caramel-colored skin and more ethnic features than my family's made me racially ambiguous.

My hair grew back after a few months, but the stress of drug dealing and running from the police continued for a few more years, until the day the feds knocked on the door of my best friend. They were looking for me about a deal gone wrong—which she immediately called to tell me. The phone call drove me on the run, and I left Seattle with two suitcases, and still estranged from my parents. They had no idea where I was or what I was involved in, other than that I was up to no good.

I flew to the Midwest to live with one of my uncles, whom I was close to, and began life anew, in my late twenties and yet emotionally still a teen. A lawyer helped clear my case, and that's all it took for me to reconsider the extreme death-defying risks I'd taken. I left it all behind: the drugs, drinking, ex-cons, and thugs, and I stayed in the Midwest until I moved to live in Tokyo for a few years.

My new self gravitated to dance and the arts, and a new crowd of friends, mostly dancers and actors and a few hairstylists.

As I tried to figure out who I was and what to do with my life, the issue of hair kept coming up. Mine was still shoulder length and wavy. In dance classes, I pulled it back into a ponytail. For the nightlife, I gooped it up with hair product.

I could see that hair was more than just a physical style. It's identity. So when the "I'm not good enough" swept through me—because "my hair isn't curly enough" or "it's too straight" or "it's too black and I wish I were blond"—I turned to my friends in the hair business for a makeover. I'd hang around the guys in my favorite salon, and they cropped my hair short, then bleached the black out so the color du jour would take hold.

My friends in the salon also got me a few jobs modeling

for print. I didn't mind all the attention this brought to my hair, but the life on parade and in the public view made my other insecurities ramp up, especially about my light brown skin color. So I lightened it with temporary skin bleaches and creams, trying to escape my multiracial looks.

The money from modeling was good and the hair products that came with the jobs were great: oils, straighteners, relaxers, shampoo, conditioner, gel and spray, mousse, tonic for hair growing, softener, thickener, tools and serum to texturize, shine, unwave, unfrizz, or volumize—especially when I bleached my black hair in blond streaks or dyed one side orange. Back then, fuchsia was my look for springtime.

My family and I had reunited by now, the adoption turmoil mostly in the past. Still, I hadn't told them I knew about my prison birth. When I summoned the courage to tell my mother that I knew about my prison roots, she said, "Oh, Deb, we were afraid to tell you, afraid what it might do to you."

My first thought forced me to bite my lip: Well, look what happened when I eventually found out.

But I kept that private. I knew she'd done the best she could and just didn't know how to break such tough information to her daughter.

Whenever my mother and I visited each other, her eyes widened when I'd show up with a new hair color. Still, we'd grown close and the steel lock on my heart had melted into the deepest of mother-daughter love.

### 3.

A new season of life, a dying parent, my mother adoptive has run out of options for staying alive. Chemo, radiation, they bought her some time but not enough. She is pushing eighty and I'm in my thirties.

I run my fingers through her chemo-thinned silver hair, but in the mother–adult daughter world of love, time wasn't on our side. There's never enough time for love.

She's in her last inhalation.

I run my fingers through her chemo-thinned silver hair.

My other hand on her shoulder, then her back.

Stroke the cotton bathrobe where my fingertips bump over her ribs.

She's in her low deep gurglegasp, the final of her breaths.

And I run my hand through her hair.

One last time.

The intimacy blends my two mothers—my hands stroking my dying mother's hair, and the strands of my baby hair that my birth mother kept.

THE STORY OF my two mothers and my hair does not end there. Not long after my mother died, I tested positive for hepatitis C, a viral disease that leads to inflammation of the liver. It's a virus transmitted by blood, sometimes from sharing needles, which I did when I injected drugs. On rare occasions, hepatitis C is passed from an intravenous-drug-using mother, like mine, to her baby. It's also rare, though, for a baby to be born in prison.

Hepatitis C can lie dormant for years, as in my case. When I learned that more Americans now die of hepatitis C than from HIV, I looked into treatment, and the most common treatment was injections of interferon over a span of a year or more. I shook my head. Not for me. I felt fine, had no symptoms that I knew about other than fatigue—but I was the mother of two children, one still a toddler, and what mother isn't exhausted?

Instead, I took the path of healthy diet and general all-around good care of myself. I'd already quit drinking, and lucky for that, because alcohol is lethal for a diseased liver. The side effects of interferon are similar to chemo: flu-like feeling, fever, chills, weight loss, nausea and vomiting, diarrhea, aches and pains, headache, poor appetite, fatigue, depression, dizziness, sore throat and mouth sores, insomnia, itching, confusion, excessive sleepiness, memory loss, and

> *The intimacy blends my two mothers—my hands stroking my dying mother's hair, and the strands of my baby hair that my birth mother kept.*

low blood counts, because white and red blood cells and platelets may temporarily decrease, putting one at increased risk for infection, anemia, and/or bleeding. It's like the pharmaceutical television ads where the glowing benefit of the drug shrinks in the long lineup of hideous side effects.

And interferon can also wreak havoc with hair: cause changes in texture and color, and hair loss, not falling in clumps, as in cancer chemo, but turning brittle and breaking off.

Here it was again, a threat to the tumble and mop of my thick, now all-black-again mop. But mostly, I didn't see the trade-off: a 20 percent chance of ridding myself of the virus with that litany of side effects. As for the hair loss, hair grows back. Liver is life. Better to lose hair than my liver.

I have a plan if I ever pursue the interferon treatment. If my hair falls out, I can follow the practice of ancient warriors. In medieval times, they used shorn hair for catapult ropes. Centuries later, they used hair for bomb fuses. This entranced me when I read about it. I've been a bomb fuse most of my life, maybe because I was born into all the ferocity and fierceness that comes with prison. Or maybe I was born not just with the wild hair but with the boldness of Medusa, though it took so many years to see and such a long time to embrace.

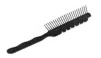

# Much Ado about Hairdos

SIRI HUSTVEDT

**W**hen my daughter was in elementary school, she wore her hair long, and every night before I began reading aloud to her, I sat behind her to comb and then braid it. If left loose during her hours of hectic sleep and dreams, Sophie's hair was transformed into a great bird's nest by morning. I especially liked the braiding ritual, liked the sight of my child's ears and the back of her neck, liked the feel and look and smell of her shiny brown hair, liked the folding over and under of the three skeins of hair between my fingers. The braiding was also an act of anticipation—it came just before we crawled into her bed together and settled in among the pillows and sheets and I began to read and Sophie to listen.

Even this simple act of plaiting my child's hair gives rise to questions about meaning. Why do more girl children wear their hair long in our culture than boy children? Why is hairstyle a sign of sexual difference? I have to admit that unless a boy child of mine had begged me for braids, I probably would have followed convention and kept his hair short, even though I think such rules are arbitrary and constricting. And finally, why would I have been mortified to send Sophie off to school with her tresses in high-flying, ratted knots?

*I especially liked the braiding ritual, liked the sight of my child's ears and the back of her neck, liked the feel and look and smell of her shiny brown hair, liked the folding over and under of the three skeins of hair between my fingers.*

All mammals have hair. Hair is not a body part so much as a lifeless extension of a body. Although the bulb of the follicle is alive, the hair shaft is dead and insensible, which allows for its multiple manipulations. We are the only mammals who braid, knot, powder, pile up, oil, spray, tease, perm, color, curl, straighten, augment, shave off, and clip our hair. The liminal status of hair is crucial to its meanings. It grows on the border between person and world. As Mary Douglas argued in *Purity and Danger*, substances that cross the body's boundaries are signs of disorder and may easily become pollutants. Hair attached to our heads is one thing, but hair clogged in the shower drain after a shampoo is waste.

Hair protrudes from all over human skin except the soles of our feet and the palms of our hands. Contiguity plays a role in hair's significance. Hair on a person's head frames her or his face, and the face is the primary focus in most of our communicative dealings with others. We recognize people by their faces. We speak, listen, nod, and respond to a face, especially to eyes. Head hair and more intrusively beard hair exist at the periphery of these vital exchanges that begin immediately after birth, and once we become self-conscious, our concern that our hair is "in place," "unmussed," or "mussed in just the right way" has to do with its role as messenger to the other.

*We are the only mammals who braid, knot, powder, pile up, oil, spray, tease, perm, color, curl, straighten, augment, shave off, and clip our hair.*

A never-combed head of hair may announce that its owner lives outside human society altogether—is a wild child, a hermit, or an insane person. It may also signify beliefs and political or cultural marginality. Think of the dreadlocks of Rastafarians or the long, matted hair of the sannyasis, ascetic wanderers in India. The combed-out Afro or "natural" for women and men in the 1960s communicated a wordless but potent political story. As a high school student, I thought of Angela Davis's hair as a sign, not only of her politics, but of her formidable intellect, as if her association with Herbert Marcuse and the Frankfurt School could be divined in her commanding halo. Was the brilliant Davis a subliminal influence on my decision in the middle of the 1970s to apply a toxic permanent wave solution to my straight, shoulder-length blond hair, a chemical alteration that was literally hair-raising? The Afro style (sort of) on me—not just a white girl, but an extremely white girl—turned the "natural" into the "unnatural." I was hardly alone in adopting the look. As fashions travel from one person or group to another, their significance mutates. Note the bleached blond hair of famous black sports stars or the penchant for cornrows among certain white people.

Despite its important role as speechless social messenger, hair is a part of the human body we can live without. Losing a head of hair or shaving our legs and underarms or waxing away pubic hair is not like losing an arm or a finger. "It will always grow back" is a phrase routinely used to comfort those who have suffered a bad haircut.

*As a high school student, I thought of Angela Davis's hair as a sign, not only of her politics, but of her formidable intellect, as if her association with Herbert Marcuse and the Frankfurt School could be divined in her commanding halo.*

Hair that touches a living head but is itself dead has an object-like quality no other body part has, except our fingernails and toenails. Hair is at once of "me" and an alien "it." When I touch the hair of another person, I am similarly touching him or her, but not his or her internally *felt* body.

I remember that when my niece Juliette was a baby, she used to suck on her bottle twirling her mother's long hair around her fingers as her eyes slowly opened and closed. It was a gesture of luxurious, soporific pleasure. Well after her bottle had been abandoned, she was unable to fall asleep without the ritual hair twiddling, which meant, of course, that the rest of my sister was forced to accompany those essential strands. Asti's hair, as part of Juliette's mother but not her mother's body proper, became what D. W. Winnicott called a "transitional object," the stuffed animal, bit of blanket, lullaby, or routine many children need to pave the way to sleep. The thing or act belongs to Winnicott's "intermediate area of experience," a between zone that is "outside the individual" but is not "the external world," an object or ritual imbued with the child's longings and fantasies that helps ease her separation from her mother. Hair as marginalia lends itself particularly well to this transitional role.

Every infant is social from birth, and without crucial interactions with an intimate caretaker, it will grow up to be severely disabled. Although the parts of the brain that control autonomic functions are quite mature at birth, emotional responses, language, and cognition develop through experience with others, and those experiences are physiologically coded in brain and body. The lullabies, head and hair stroking, rocking, cooing, playing, talk, and babble that take place between parent and baby during infancy are accompanied by synaptic brain connectivity unique to a particular individual. The cultural-social is not a category that hovers over the physical; it becomes the physical body itself. Human perception develops through a dynamic learning process, and when perceptual, cognitive, and motor skills are learned well enough, they become automatic and unconscious—part of implicit memory. It is when automatic perceptual patterns are interrupted by a novel experience, however, that we require full consciousness to reorder our expectation, be it about hair or anything else.

When Sophie went off to school with her two long, neat braids swinging behind her, she did not disturb anyone's expectations, but when the psychologist Sandra Bem sent her four-year-old boy, Jeremy, off to nursery school wearing the barrettes he had requested she put in his hair, he was hounded by a boy in his class who kept insisting that "only girls wear barrettes." Jeremy sensibly replied that barrettes don't matter. He had a penis and testicles and this fact made him a boy, not a girl. His classmate, however, remained unconvinced, and in a moment of exasperation, Jeremy pulled down his pants to give proof of his boyhood. After a quick glance, his comrade said, "Everybody has a penis. Only girls wear barrettes." Most boys in contemporary Western culture begin to resist objects, colors, and hairdos coded as feminine as soon as they have become certain of their sexual identity, around the age of three. Jeremy's fellow pupil seems to have been muddled about penises and vulvas, but adamant about social convention. In this context, the barrette metamorphosed from innocuous hair implement to an object of gender subversion. The philosopher Judith Butler would call Jeremy's barrette-wearing a kind of "performativity," gender as doing, not being.

Girls have more leeway to explore masculine forms than boys. Unlike barrettes on a boy, short hair on a girl is not subject to ridicule, noteworthy because the "feminine" has far more polluting power for a boy in our culture than the "masculine" has for a girl. During three or four years before she reached puberty, another niece of mine, Ava, had a short haircut and was sometimes identified as a boy. One year she played with gender performance in the costume she chose for Halloween: half of her went as a girl, the other half as a boy. Hair was a vital element in this down-the-middle disguise. The long flowing locks of a wig adorned the girl half. Her own short hair served the boy half.

I began the fifth grade with long hair, but at some point in the middle of the year I chopped it into what was then called a pixie cut. When I returned to school newly shorn, I was informed that the boy I *liked*, a boy who had supposedly *liked me back*, had withdrawn his affection. It had been swept away and discarded at the hairdresser's along with my silky locks. I recall thinking that my former admirer was a superficial twit, but perhaps he had succumbed to a Goldilocks fantasy. He would not be the last male personage in my life to fixate on feminine blondness and its myriad associations in our culture, including abstract qualities such as purity, innocence, stupidity, childishness, and sexual allure embodied by multiple figures—the goddesses Sif and Freya and the Valkyries of Norse mythology, the multitudes of fair maidens in fairy tales, numerous heroines in Victorian novels and melodramas, and cinematic bombshells, such as Harlow and Monroe (both of whom I love to watch on-screen). The infantile and dumb connotations of *blond* may explain why I have often dreamed of a buzz cut. The fairy-tale and mythological creatures so dear to me as a child may explain why I have had short hair as an adult but never *that* short and did not turn myself into a brunette or redhead. A part of me must hesitate to shear myself of all blond, feminine meanings, as if next to no hair would mean severing a connection to an earlier self.

Iris, the narrator of my first novel, *The Blindfold*, crops her hair during a period in her life of defensive transformation. She wanders around New York City after dark wearing a man's suit. She gives herself the name of a sadistic boy in a German novel she has translated: Klaus.

> The gap between what I was forced to acknowledge to the world— namely, that I was a woman—and what I dreamed inwardly didn't bother me. By becoming Klaus at night I had effectively blurred my gender. The suit, my clipped head and unadorned face

altered the world's view of who I was, and I became someone else through its eyes. I even spoke differently as Klaus. I was less hesitant, used more slang, and favored colorful verbs.

My heroine's butch haircut partakes of her second act of translation, from feminine Iris to masculine Klaus, a performance that belies the notion that appearance is purely superficial. By playing with her hair and clothes, she subverts cultural expectations that have shaped her in ways she finds demeaning.

Short hair or long? Interpretations of length change with time and place. The Merovingian kings (ca. 457–750) wore their hair long as a sign of their high status. Samson's strength famously resided in his hair. The composer Franz Liszt's shoulder-length hair became the object of frenzied, fetishistic female desire. The mini narratives of television commercials for formulas to cure male baldness reinforce the notion that the fluff above is linked to action below. Once a man's hair has been miraculously restored, a seductive woman inevitably appears beside him on the screen to caress his newly sprouted locks. But then shampoo commercials for women also contain sexual messages that long, and sometimes short, frequently windblown tresses will enchant a dream man.

Because of its proximity to adult genitals, pubic hair is bound to have special meanings. Turkish women, for example, remove their pubic hair. In a paper on the meanings of hair in Turkey, the anthropologist Carol Delaney reported that during a visit to a public bath for a prenuptial ritual, the soon-to-be bride advised her to bathe before the other women so they would not see her "like a goat." The expression moves us from the human to the bestial. Metaphor is the way the human mind travels. As George Lakoff and Mark Johnson argued in their landmark book *Metaphors We Live By*, "spatialization metaphors are rooted in physical and cultural experience." Head hair is *up* on the body; pubic hair is *down*. Humans are *superior* to animals. Reason is a *higher* function; emotions are *lower* ones. Men are associated with the intellect—head—and women with passion—genitals. Hair *above* can be flaunted; hair *below* must be concealed and sometimes removed altogether.

Sigmund Freud's brief interpretation of Medusa (1922) with her decapitated head, snaky mane, and petrifying gaze operates through a down-up movement. For Freud, the mythical Gorgon's head represented a boy's castration fears upon seeing "the female genitals, probably those of an adult, surrounded by hair, and essentially those of the mother." The source of terror (the threatened penis) migrates upward and is turned into a maternal head with phallic serpents instead of hair. The horrible countenance makes the boy stiff with fear, a rigid state that nevertheless consoles him because it signifies an erection (my penis is still here). Indeed, Jeremy's classmate, whose anatomical beliefs were predicated on the idea of a universal penis, might have been stunned by a girl with no feminine accoutrements, no barrettes, to signal girlness, and no penis to boot. Would the child have felt his own member was threatened by the revelation? There have been countless critiques of Freud's brief sketch, as well as revisionist readings of the mythical Gorgon, including Hélène Cixous's feminist manifesto: "The Laugh of the Medusa."

What interests me here is the part of the story Freud suppresses. The mother's vulva, *surrounded by hair*, is the external sign of a hidden origin, our first residence in utero, the place from which we were all expelled during the contractions of labor and birth. Isn't this bit of anatomical news also startling for children? Phallic sexuality is clearly involved in the Medusa myth, and the snake as an image for male sexuality is hardly limited to the Western tradition. (In Taipei in 1975, I watched a man slice open a snake and drink its blood to enhance his potency.) The Medusa story exists in several versions, but it always includes intercourse—Poseidon's dalliance with or rape of Medusa, and subsequent births. In Ovid, after Perseus beheads the Gorgon, her drops of blood give birth to Chrysaor, a young man, and Pegasus, the mythical winged horse. In other versions, the offspring emerge from the Gorgon's neck. Either way, the myth includes a monstrous but fecund maternity.

Hair has and continues to have sexual meanings, although whether there is any universal quality to them is a matter of debate. In his famous 1958 essay "Magical Hair," the anthropologist Edmund Leach developed a cross-cultural formula: "Long hair = unrestrained sexuality; short hair or partially shaved head or tightly bound hair = restricted sexuality; closely shaved head = celibacy." Leach was deeply influenced by Freud's thoughts on phallic heads, although for him hair sometimes played an ejaculatory role as emanating semen. No doubt phallic significance has accumulated around hair in many cultures, but the persistent adoption of an exclusively male perspective (everybody has a penis) consistently fails to see meanings that are ambiguous, multilayered, and hermaphroditic, not either/or, but both-and.

One of the many tales I loved as a child and read to Sophie after our hair-braiding ritual was "Rapunzel." The Grimm story has multiple sources, including the tenth-century Persian tale of Rudaba, from the epic poem *Shannameh*, in which the heroine offers the hero her long, dark tresses as a rope to climb (he refuses because he is afraid to hurt her), and the medieval legend of Saint Barbara, in which the pious girl is locked in a tower by her brutal father, a story that Christine de Pisan retells in *The Book of the City of Ladies* (1405), her great work written to protest misogyny. The later tales "Petrosinella" (1634) by Giambattista Basile and "Persinette" (1698) by Charlotte Rose de Caumont de la Force are much closer to the Grimm version (1812), which the brothers adopted from the German writer Friedrich Schultz (1790).

In all the last four versions of the tale, the action begins with a pregnant woman's cravings for an edible plant (rampion, parsley, lettuce, or a kind of radish—rapunzel) that grows in a neighboring garden owned by a powerful woman (enchantress, sorceress, ogress, or witch). The husband steals the forbidden plant for his wife, is caught, and, to avoid punishment for his crime, promises his neighbor the unborn child. The enchantress keeps the girl locked in a high tower but comes and goes by climbing her captive's long hair, which then becomes the vehicle for the prince's clandestine entrance to the tower. The final Grimm version, cleansed for its young audience, does not include Rapunzel's swelling belly or the birth of twins, but "Petrosinella" and "Persinette" do. When the enchantress realizes the girl is pregnant, she flies into a rage, chops off the offending hair, and uses it as a lure to trap the unsuspecting lover. The heroine and hero are separated, suffer and pine for each other, but are eventually reunited.

Rapunzel's fantastical head of hair figures as an intermediate zone where both unions and separations are enacted. A pregnancy begins the story, after all, and the lifeline between mother and fetus is the umbilical cord, cut after birth. But an infant's dependence on her mother does not end with this anatomical separation. Rapunzel's hair or extensive braid is a vehicle by which the mother-witch figure comes and goes on her visits, an apt metaphor for the back-and-forth motion, presence and absence of the mother for the child that Freud famously elaborated in *Beyond the Pleasure Principle* when he described his one-and-a-half-year-old grandson playing with a spool and string. The little boy casts out his string, accompanied by a long

"oooo," which his mother interpreted as his attempt to say
"*fort*," gone, after which he reels it in and joyfully says "*da*,"
there. The game is one of magically mastering the painful
absence of the mother, and the string, which Freud does not
talk about, serves as the sign or symbol of the relation: I am
connected to you. Rapunzel's hair, then, is a sign of evolving
human passions, first for the mother, then for the grown-up
love object and the phallic/vaginal fusion between lovers that
returns us to the story's beginning: a woman finds herself in
the plural state of pregnancy.

The story's form is circular, not linear, and its narrative excitement turns on violent cuts: the infant is forcibly removed
from her mother at birth, then locked in a tower, cut off from
others, and jealously guarded by the story's second, postpar-
tum maternal figure. After the punishing haircut, Rapunzel
is not only estranged from her lover, she loses the sorceress
mother. Notably, Charlotte Rose de Caumont de la Force
reconciles the couple and the enchantress in "Persinette," an
ending that is not only satisfying but one that dramatizes the
fact that this is a tale of familial struggles.

A child's early sociopsychobiological bond with and dependence on her mother changes over time. Maternal love
may be ferocious, ecstatic, covetous, and resistant to intrud-
ers, including the child's father and later the offspring's love
objects, but if all goes well the mother accepts her child's

independence. She lets her go. Rapunzel's long hair, which belongs to her, but which may be hacked off without injuring her, is the perfect metaphor for the transitional space in which the passionate and sometimes tortured connections and separations between mother and child happen. And it is in this same space of back-and-forth exchanges that a baby's early babbling becomes first comprehensible speech and then narrative, a symbolic communicative form that links, weaves, and spins words into a structural whole with a beginning, a middle, and an end, one that can summon what used to be, what might be, or what could never be. Rapunzel's supernaturally long cord of hair that yokes one person to another may be assigned yet another metaphorical meaning—it is a trope for the telling of the fairy tale itself.

My daughter is grown up. I remember combing and braiding her hair, and I remember reading her stories, stories that still live between us, stories that used to soothe her into sleep.

# Two Hair Stories from One Life

. . . . . . . . . . . . . . . . . . . . . . . . . . . . . . . . . . . . . . . . . . . . . .

## MYRA GOLDBERG

"Think about what you're *really* interested in," I told the writing class. "As opposed to what you *should* be interested in." This was an evening writing class of grown women. We had a retired surgeon, a man, but he quit when we didn't accept him as an authority on anything but medicine. It was the 1980s. I don't remember why I asked them this question. Only that I'd been struck when a friend quoted her friend's question: "Do you want to know what I think? Or do you want to know what I *really* think?"

Writing, I thought, is what you *really* think. And what you really want to think about. "I'm interested in hair, for example," I said to my students. "I sit on the subway and plan new hairdos for people. Also, I keep track of my students' constantly changing hairdos."

Everyone started talking at once to her neighbors, telling stories. They stayed late. The next class, I brought a tape recorder.

"Hair," I said. "We're going to go back to talking about hair." Everyone was enthusiastic. I was exhausted by the time this class met. I taught undergraduates at Sarah Lawrence all day, then made extra money with classes like this one. For most of these women, it was a time to be with other adults and free of their kids, free to find out what they really thought. I had no kids but had bought an apartment in preparation for one. "Get a piece of the rock first," a friend had advised.

"Hair? Like on our heads?" asked the woman who'd missed the last session.

"Oh, absolutely." I told them a version of my own life lessons in hair: Learning to make a pageboy (seventh grade), Audrey Hepburn's bangs (eighth grade), a dancer's bun until junior year, then something tousled through college. Long, straight, center-parted hair until I noticed that most of the woman on the pro-choice march on Washington had the same hairdo. Each change promised more than it delivered. I would be a different person with my new do, I felt when young. I would feel different but be the same person, I felt later. People would regard me differently with a new hairdo, so I would feel different inside, still later on. At last, I settled for looking a little different, but not much. Hair became hair, not transformation.

"I've been thinking about hair since this group met," I told them. "I went home last week and said to the man I live with, 'Oh, we had this wonderful meeting, we accidentally started talking about hair at the end. Now we're going to talk about it next week.' I could tell by the quality of his silence that he couldn't hear what I was saying, which made me tongue tied."

"I've got a hair story, if you want one," said a woman who rarely spoke in class. "I'm thinking that maybe I'm going to get my hair cut. That's my only story about hair. Also, when my grandmother came to this country—she got married, you know, over there, and all her beautiful hair got cut off, which was what those Jews in Europe did. But secretly, she knew she was coming here, so she grew it a little under the wig. And when she saw that Statue of Liberty, she took off her wig with her children beside her and threw it into the harbor. After that she never cut her hair. Her hair was black and long. My grandfather brushed it. Everybody brushed her hair."

"My aunt always wore a turban," said our neurologist. "I thought she was bald. Nowadays I'd think that turban was East African, Caribbean, but this was Atlanta in the nineteen fifties. Anyway, we had this box of photographs at home, and one day

I found her there, with this gorgeous skin and coppery hair, ringlets. Good hair, in the parlance. 'Did she have a sickness?' I asked my mama. 'Hiding that hair?'"

"Also, when you were talking about language," said the woman who rarely spoke. "I don't speak hair language: layers and blunt cuts and so on. At the beauty parlor, they want to know in that language what you want them to do to you. My husband says unless I know the language of each trade, all I can do is submit to them."

"What else can you do?"

"Insist on something you can't describe," said the neurologist with the aunt from Atlanta. "Or use pictures, from those magazines."

"My mother, from the time I was seven or eight, was absolutely obsessed about her hair." A teacher from Queens. "Which I now realize she must have communicated internal states of being through, which I didn't think she had. My mother—not that I blame her—growing up in the most banal and horrible Irish poverty, will not spend more than twelve dollars for a haircut."

"Where does she get them?"

"Astoria."

"My mother, the only negative comment she'll make about people directly is about hair. She wouldn't go around to my brother's house in Atlanta and say you dress terribly, but she will tell him he needs a haircut."

And so we moved from hair to hair and mothers, which turns out to be a topic grown women have a lot to say about. My mother's hair, like mine, and like her mother's, grew in wavy circles, which made it easily cut into something tousled, but too wavy for a proper American flip, pageboy, or shag. My mother's mother came from Russia as an anarchist and became a suffragette here, taking wages from my grandfather, when she worked in their store, and saving them so my aunts and mother could go to college. "I want my girls to be accomplished," she said, and they were accomplished, a writer, a painter, and a translator. They carried a European disapproval of excessive interest in one's looks, along with a belief in yogurt, Russian literature, social justice, and exercise, from one generation to another. For me to suggest this frivolous topic for a class was a departure from my family's values.

As it turned out, I made a written collage from the tape, then a theater piece, performed at Sarah Lawrence, then downtown, then in DC, in a theater festival, where the comedienne before me sat drinking beer on a toilet seat and nobody in the drunk and disorderly audience seemed interested in hair that night. As if to honor the values of my mother and grandmother, I'd sprinkled the piece with references to slavery and language, as if I were showing how big, how not trivial, the subject was. At that point in history, *feminine* was still a synonym for *trivial*. I'd had my own nontrivial experience with hair in Japan.

"In Hiroshima," I told the women, "where I went on a trip,

there was this sign in this museum. JAPANESE WOMEN VALUE THEIR BLACK HAIR. This is the atom bomb museum, and the picture here is of a woman with most of her scalp bare. I stared and I stared. Her whole life is ruined, I thought, no one will marry her and she can never have children. Then something American, tastelessly pragmatic, but smart, came over me. Why doesn't she just forget her shame and buy a wig, for God's sake, I thought, and get on with her life and solve her problems?"

I said that. I felt that. At that time, my own problem was a yearning for a child, so I took my own advice and adopted a daughter.

AND THAT WAS that for hair, for a while. Writing can take what is obsessive, conflicted, or riveting and put it behind you. Hair dropped into the category of the familiar itch. I noticed hairdos and inquired after the hairdressers who'd done them. But hair was definitely the background music to my life with my daughter, whose birth mother's hair was blond and straight and whose African American father, who was in the air force, had a buzz cut. He was married with kids. She was eighteen and looked like an Appalachian Virgin Mary when she handed Anna to me in the chapel, and I looked like a sympathetic, Semitic, guilty, older arty type, in a quilted fake Appalachian jacket. Anna looked like a large, beautiful baby doll.

Before adopting, when I mentioned difficulties I might face raising a biracial child, people often started talking about hair. I thought that was silly. How hard could doing a kid's hair be? In fact, the actual doing of the hair was less difficult than the reception we got for her hair. This is like race, which Americans tend to think of as skin color, or mean words, or something from the past, rather than as a system and history in which some people are rewarded and others held back. Meanwhile, like it or not, we all operate within a system. Our system was a visually different mother and daughter. If I could wear my hair tousled and rough cut, Anna could not. When I made her fat braids like Pippi Longstocking's, they would damage her self-esteem, according to her white pre-K teacher. Her halo of curls was too boyish, according to a neighbor. Nobody had told my mother what to do with my hair. But instead of staring them down, I looked for someone knowledgeable to guide me and found Madeline, a fabulous teenager from a Dominican family. Dominicans are New York City's best hairdressers these days. They come in all skin colors and hair types and know how to do the hair of girls like Anna, a Mixed Chick, according to her shampoo bottle.

Watching Madeline do Anna's hair, I could see I was unable

> *Before adopting, when I mentioned difficulties I might face raising a biracial child, people often started talking about hair.*

to let Anna scream for the sake of a smooth crown and a tight ponytail. Apparently, excessively tight-pulled hair, by my standards, was bottom-line respectability for hair like Anna's. So Madeline did Anna's hair, and I helped with Madeline's college essays and applications. Meanwhile, Anna would stay over at Madeline's family's house, and they would all take care pulling and combing and washing and listening to her scream. When she returned, she looked like a proper what? Dominican? Black girl? Biracial daughter of a white mother?

When Madeline got placed on the waiting list at Mount Holyoke, I wrote a letter for her. I mentioned my position as a professor at a sisterly school. I mentioned her resourcefulness, intelligence, and fortitude. I did not mention that she knew what to do with my daughter's hair. Mount Holyoke took her and her skills. She went on to become a doctor, a PhD, and a mother of three. I got left alone with Anna's hair just as she entered kindergarten. Then the chair of my department, a close friend, died, and I took over his responsibilities at work.

Once or twice, in my grief and distraction, I noticed Anna scratching her head but thought nothing of it. There was a lice epidemic in the kindergarten class, and a distraught mother spread the rumor that the epidemic was Anna's fault. (These epidemics run through early childhood. Who starts them is impossible to trace. God, maybe.) The angry mother went to the principal and suggested they call the Bureau of Child Welfare on us. Another former student called to warn me. An African American mother called too. "Lice don't like our hair," she said, meaning her and Anna's hair, no doubt. "They don't like the oils we use." But I didn't use these oils on Anna's hair.

Then she added, "But you really must do something about that hair."

I hired an Orthodox Jewish nitpicker to pick the nits out. I poured olive oil over Anna's head to get rid of whatever the nitpicker had used. I found a Dominican salon, which cut off a lot of her hair. I took Anna to FAO Schwarz to make up for the loss of her hair and bought her a doll and doll carriage. Earlier on, we had both considered FAO Schwarz a museum instead of a store. The distraught mother told people not to invite Anna to their children's birthday parties. Another, a therapist, jostled Anna when she came into the kindergarten class.

By now, I felt I lacked a lot more than hair skills. I felt I'd missed the part of life—was it in seventh grade?—where you learned to defend yourself. I couldn't defend my child or teach her how to be the kind of person who didn't get messed with. Maybe African American mothers were braiding that kind of knowledge into their daughters' heads.

I blamed my high-minded family, who thought you should

rise above petty insults and focus on the big picture, whatever that was. Then I met with the teacher and the principal,
whose reception was lukewarm and who promised no help.
At the end of the year, I moved Anna to a self-consciously
integrated private school, where the parents were better be-
haved, mostly. By now, I can see that people are often at their
worst in the midst of child rearing.

WHEN ANNA REACHED high school, she did her
own hair, did it beautifully, and went back to public school.
There were other issues. The black kids thought she was rich,
and the white kids admired her for being ghetto. A former
friend pushed her down the school stairs, then threatened to
have her boyfriend bring his gang around. The girl's boyfriend was a drug dealer. I went to the principal about the
staircase incident and the threat. He was noncommittal. If
in the earlier hair incident I felt the teacher and principal
were confused about this odd couple, mother and daughter, I
now felt this man considered Anna overprivileged, compared
to her friend. It was Anna's friend who needed his help, he
signaled. We were on our own.

"Tell Natasha, if her boyfriend touches you, I'll drop a
dime on him," I told Anna. I had learned this line from a
hippie relative with experience in the drug trade.

"Oh, is that how we do it?" she said. It's hard to express
the emotion in this exchange, as if Anna had been waiting

her whole life to find out how people like us stood up for themselves. We didn't get into fistfights or join gangs. I barely had the time for drama. Unlike the mothers of some of her friends, I didn't say, I'll kill that kid when she gets home. Once, I had taken her iPod away as a punishment but felt ridiculous. Now, making this threat, I knew I wouldn't carry it out. I didn't believe in the drug laws. I didn't believe in the prisons. Still, a threat is valuable until it isn't.

By now, Anna's hair hung in curls around her shoulders, dark at the roots, auburn elsewhere. The hairdo was something she'd invented, neither entirely natural nor tormented. I had nothing to do with this hairdo. She had tried braids at the African braiders on 125th Street, then had her hair straightened until she looked like Diana Ross. She had been blond and black haired, austere and stylish. Now, she looked beautiful, self-assured, and expensive. If hair was a language, she was fluent in it.

A sacrament, say the Anglicans, is an outward visible sign of an inward, invisible state.

"I don't know what you should do about Natasha," I said. "You know her better than I do." I was stumped, I meant, because I knew next to nothing about the world she was in these days. I hadn't even known, as Anna once pointed out, that she was treated one way when I was with her and another when I wasn't. "I'm sure you'll figure it out," I added, and I meant that too. Look what she had figured out about her hair, I thought.

The boyfriend didn't bring his gang around. I didn't ask what threat she'd used, if any. And that was the beginning of my recognition that Anna would be able to find her own way through the world. All parents face this moment. Very few, I'm guessing, find the answer in their daughter's hair.

# Capelli Lunghi

· · · · · · · · · · · · · · · · · · · · · · · · · · · · · · · · · · · · · · · · · · · · · · · · ·

## JULIA FIERRO

**A**fter I had my three-year-old daughter's hair cut short last summer, neighbors stopped us on the street.

"What happened?" they asked in hushed incredulity, as if my little girl had broken a limb. My husband's first response to the haircut was nervous laughter, and asking me why I'd "scalped" our daughter.

Everywhere we went that summer, people commented on her lack of hair—the cashier at the pizza parlor, the crossing guard near her preschool, the owner of our neighborhood convenience store. I avoided posting photos of her on Facebook, anticipating the reaction, and when I finally did, the comments of surprise, and even accusation—*What did you do to her?*—piled one on top of the other.

*Where are her curls?*

*Did she do this to herself?!*

*She looks like a little boy* (modified with an apologetic winking smiley face emoticon).

My daughter's playmates' parents didn't recognize her at first and then acted as if they loved the change. *She's so cute, like a little hipster!* Or they seemed confused, unable to lie. *She just looks so different.* Sometimes they comforted me with a pat on the shoulder—*Don't worry, the curls could grow back.*

I smiled and laughed and shrugged my shoulders in mock bewilderment, but here's what I was really thinking: Why would I let my adorable little girl, so often compared to the dimple-cheeked, ringlet-adorned Shirley Temple, be turned into what most strangers thought was an adorable little boy?

I made excuses for what began to feel like something I'd done, a crime committed. *It was a terribly hot summer,* I said. True. *She wanted to have her hair cut short,* I explained to people who were practically strangers, feeling pressured to make my case. True. *She loves her new haircut!* Also true. She had happily squealed, *I look like a boy!* when she first studied the new do in the mirror. She loathed hair clips, headbands, and ponytails, pulling the rainbow-colored hair bands out and using them instead as slingshots for her Lego figurines. All true. So why did I feel as if I was lying to my husband when I told him, several weeks after what we were calling, half-jokingly, "the cut," that it wasn't my fault and that I blamed the stylist instead? I was distracted, I explained, I'd been watching my newly shorn six-year-old son run around the shop—*Don't touch that! Slow down! Be careful!*—and simultaneously paying for both their haircuts, while his sister sat in the raised salon chair shaped like a yellow NYC taxicab. When the hairstylist asked me how I'd like my daughter's hair cut, I'd answered, *Short is fine!* over my shoulder, not bothering to give any specific instructions.

It *was* all my fault, I thought, she *did* look like a boy. But I refused to admit this aloud. There

*Why would I let my adorable little girl, so often compared to the dimple-cheeked, ringlet-adorned Shirley Temple, be turned into what most strangers thought was an adorable little boy?*

was a bigger truth that would have been even worse to admit: I wanted her to go back to looking like a girl. The coils of blond-streaked curls had softened her features, had made her mouth a rosy little bow, her eyelashes fuller. Those ringlets had been her most feminine trait, especially for an active little girl who refused to wear dresses or any clothing that was frilly or pink. I reminded myself that I was proud of my daughter's athleticism and strength and of the fact that she loved to play in the dirt with her older brother. She was completely and confidently herself. She was everything I had *not* been allowed to be as a child, with my pink-carpeted bedroom and canopy bed, my ballet classes and taffeta holiday dresses. But after her curls were gone, I found myself missing them, even yearning for them.

Wanting my daughter to look like a girl made me feel not only like a bad mother, but also like a bad feminist. I was an open-minded, educated, modern mother, I told myself. When my son asked for a pink doll stroller, I bought it for him happily. When my daughter shook her head at the lovely dresses hanging in her closet and chose jeans and T-shirts, I gritted my teeth and acquiesced. So why would a silly haircut matter so much? Hadn't I been a little girl like my daughter once, a little girl expected to be polite and demure and graceful—feminine? Didn't I remember the weight of all that thick, glossy hair that had hung to my waist throughout my girlhood? I began to suspect that I wasn't any more enlightened a parent than my mother and father had been. This belief in my progressive and emotionally intelligent parenting philosophy had carried me through the most challenging and self-doubting moments of early motherhood, but here I was, criticizing my daughter's hair because it wasn't feminine enough.

As we drove toward my parents' suburban home for the

> *Wanting my daughter to look like a girl made me feel not only like a bad mother, but also like a bad feminist.*

first visit since "the cut," my daughter looking in the rearview mirror and happily admiring her hair, it was my father's reaction I worried about most. I'd already received, loud and clear, my mother's retort to the photos on my Facebook page, which she kept open on her computer monitor all day, hoping to catch a glimpse of her grandkids. *Her curls made her pretty, but without them she's still cute*, my mother had said, both a reprimand and a consolation. But my father wasn't interested in Facebook, and this would be the first time he'd seen the evidence of my screwup.

What if he yelled at me in front of the children? They knew him only as sweet Nonno, the grandfather who made them *pasta fagiole* and sneaked them M&M's when he thought Mommy and Daddy weren't looking; as the gentle old man they adored, who cuddled them on his lap and sang them traditional Neapolitan lullabies. They didn't know the man who had fallen into mercurial and agitated moods in my own childhood, when life in a foreign country felt wretched—the impossible language, convoluted customs, and harried pace. His dark moods had led to enraged fights with my mother, and to his promising he'd leave us and return to Italy if she continued to *throw away* money. Sometimes they led to his hitting me with his hands, his belt, and the wooden kitchen spoon and threatening a bigger punishment, which I felt even then was both ludicrous and terrifying: he threatened to hang me by my hair from a nail in the wall.

WHEN I WAS a girl, my father insisted I keep my hair long, just as generations of southern Italian women had before me, he reminded me often. *Capelli lunghi.* In the few photos I've seen of my grandmother and my aunts in their lives before America, with their solid farmers' bodies framed by the cliffs of the Amalfi Coast, their hair hangs heavy around their unsmiling faces, as though they are draped in mourning shawls.

As the first girl born into my father's family, I was treated like a treasured doll. My mother dressed me for the part—ruffled dresses and hand-knit sweaters and capes. The signoras in Turin, where we lived until I was two years old, before moving to New York, would stop my mother in the street to coo over me, fingering my lace-trimmed bloomers and shiny patent-leather shoes, and whisper, *Che bambola!* What a doll! I was doted on, especially by my uncles, both of whom had boys. If I wanted something—fresh gnocchi, a lollipop, a ride on my godfather's Vespa—my wish was their command. They called me *la principessa.* The little princess.

My hair—long, thick, a rich brown, with a subtle wave—was my most remarkable feature. My mother would smile proudly at the compliments, not mentioning the monthly trips to the beauty parlor, where two women worked in tandem to comb through the snarls as my eyes watered with pain. In my last year of elementary school, when my mother took me to the neurologist for my frequent migraines, he suggested cutting my hair. My mother refused this advice: I needed my hair, she explained. I was to play the coveted role of Clara in *The Nutcracker* that winter, and the mothers in charge of hair and makeup would use a hot iron to twist my hair into long, bouncing banana curls, which they'd spray with Aqua Net and adorn with silk bows. In my childhood, women—my mother, her friends, aunts, school friends, their mothers—loved my hair as much as men would a decade later. My hair was what made me special. My hair was my source of beauty. My power. My hair was what my daughter, who still sees the world in black-and-white terms, as *good guys* and *bad guys*, would call my "invincible shield."

When I was a sophomore in high school, my mother and the mothers of my two best friends threw us a sweet sixteen party on a boat that cruised around the Statue of Liberty. My father had fought her on the party, claiming, rightly so, that the cost was outrageous. I imagined he was thinking of his own teenage years, a glimpse of which I've seen in a single creased sepia-toned photo, where he stood alongside several stick-thin boys in front of the rocky southern Italian landscape. A rope holds his pants up. His shirt is stained. But he poses with his hands on his hips, his chin jutting forth arrogantly.

In anticipation of the party, all three of us birthday girls had picked out floral Laura Ashley dresses. My mother had used a credit card she kept from my father and insisted I keep my dress in the trunk of her car until my father went to bed. The fantasy I had of myself in my sweet sixteen dress included my first pair of high heels, a strapless bra my mother had bought me just for the occasion (although I barely needed it), and a haircut. I imagined the ends of my new short hair fluttering in the sea breeze and tickling the tops of my bare shoulders, as our birthday-boat cruise wound its way to the Statue of Liberty and back. I wanted a cute bob that would make me look, or at least feel, like Daisy in *The Great Gatsby*, which we had just read in school, and which felt dreamily fateful, since I lived on the North Shore of Long Island surrounded by attractive blue-blooded families—mothers who wore tennis skirts to school pickup, fathers who commuted to the city in three-piece suits. These were people who boated and skied and knew when plaid and floral went together, a sixth sense I imagined they were born with. My parents had moved to this affluent area so I could be raised among the rich, hoping some of the privilege would rub off on me. I worked hard to fit in, and with the help of the pricey clothes my mother bought me, I claimed a spot on the margins of the in crowd.

In retrospect, it seems ridiculous that I asked my father for permission to cut my hair when he had already said no so many times, when he was surely anxious about the money being spent on the party, a panic unique to those who know what it feels like to cry in pain from hunger. But as I've come to learn, so much of survival—for me, for my father—is about delusion. *You should have known he'd say no*, I chastise my sixteen-year-old self, blinded by an entitled sense of want and hope, like a naïve Juliet. I should have foreseen his response—his eyes growing impossibly large, his running after me with an open hand, reaching for and yanking my long hair, which flew behind me like reins meant for his grip. Then he was hitting me and I moved to that space (inside myself? above myself?) where I was both present and not, where time moved both slowly and quickly, where sound became dull, like the ticking of a watch wrapped in cotton, and when I returned to the present, my father was gone, the tracks of his feet in the shag carpet, the sunlit room filled with the frenzied dance of dust motes, welts on my arms and legs—*nothing major*, I thought—and I went to the kitchen where he was sitting at the table and crying, and I forgave him, made him promise he wouldn't kill himself or something stupid like that. And I promised him I would keep my hair long.

WHEN WE ARRIVED at my parents' house, my shorn daughter skipped up the front steps and into my father's arms. Once we were inside the house, it was my mother who had the strongest reaction to "the cut." *You cut away her personality!* I could feel my father nearby. What would he say? What would he do?

As I launched into the string of excuses and tried to explain to my mother that her granddaughter was delighted to look just like her hero, her big brother, I prepared myself for my father's anger—the literal darkening of his face, the deepening of his voice, the Neapolitan curses he used in only the most incensed moments.

"Looks good," my father said. *"Insieme."*

The same.

He pointed to my daughter's head and then to my own head. My daughter and I had the same boy's haircut. I'd had my own hair cut short when I turned twenty, after I'd been living on my own for three years. And when my father had first seen my new stylish pixie cut, during one of my rare visits back home, he had admired it and said I looked *sophisticated.* All those times we'd fought over my hair, whether with words or with his open hands, the battle had been about so much more than hair: for me, independence; for him, a kind of warped protection of me and a grasping for the control he couldn't find in the foreign world outside our home's walls. And here he was now, an old man, at the end of his life, filled with his own private fears and regrets, but also love—for my daughter and, through her, for me. I forgave him, again.

I'm STILL NOT sure what happened that day at the kids' hair salon. Had I meant to have my daughter's lovely curlicues cut away? They were the feature that had led so many people—sometimes strangers on the street—to peer into her dimple-cheeked face and compare her to Shirley Temple, my mother's childhood idol and a figure I had felt, consciously or not, was a model for me as a girl. She was—I was—a little princess who kept her chin up no matter how bleak her life, no matter how many times my father, whom I love, threatened to hang me by my hair from a nail in the wall. It had been a threat I did not wholly believe, but I also could not dismiss it as silly or idle. Was I still haunted by it? Even a little? Maybe that fine balance—the small but terrifying possibility I'd grown up with—had been with me the day my daughter's curls fell to the floor. Or was it only the buried memory of my fear that had made her haircut so difficult for me to ignore?

# Heavy Mettle

· · · · · · · · · · · · · · · · · · · · · · · · · · · · · · · · · · · · · · · · · · ·

## DEBORAH HOFMANN

When I was growing up, my mother often told me that in my high chair I smeared oatmeal and mashed potatoes into my hair and that she could see that this was an expression of pure bliss. When the messy meal was over, she would hoist me to the sink for cleanup, a ritual of splashes and giggles. Part of the story she told is that I was a butterball of an infant and that she, suffering from a starving marriage, was emaciated, weighing at times barely ninety pounds. In the wake of her marital misery, these sessions provided a mutually nourishing understanding that my hair was also hers and that it was a source of pleasure and connection.

From about four to seven, I was skinny and I had scabs capping my knees, but my real trademark was my elegant waist-long brown braid. Mommy genuinely believed that cutting hair like mine was akin to desecration, like defiling nature or art. Trimming my split ends pained her, so she usually talked herself out of it. No pigtails or ponytails; those hurt, from all the yanking and tight rubber bands, and they were far too closely suggestive of the trophy squirrel tails many of our neighbors in rural Illinois with BB guns customized as bicycle handle ornaments. After my parents divorced, we were poor, and on top of that burden, we paid for water. To save money, some nights my little brother and I had baths one after the other, in the same water.

*My hair, like a Persian rug, she said, was my own magic flying carpet. Adventures and romance would be mine. Taking care of my hair seemed part of the fare.*

On such evenings before a bath, or on Saturday mornings, I could be found pumping myself on a creaking swing. My mother would unfurl my rope of a braid and let it cascade in long, rippling strands. I would again indulge in the deliberate messing of my hair in the pursuit of ecstasy. As I gained liftoff from the earth below and pumped the blue sky to go higher, higher, higher, I would lean back and let my hair leave sweeping contrails in the dirt as my feet touched the clouds. And my mother's shampooing it in the bathtub later and asking about my playtime—that was an indoor encounter with heavenly innocent security, and a prelude to bedtime prayers.

I swanned into Sunday school with soft banana curls after Mommy poised me on a stool to unwind strips of roller rags. Her scolding, "Debbieleine, sit still, please," worked momentarily. But I never could resist a wriggle to look off to the side at Captain Kangaroo on television. Like mine, his bangs were so crooked. Clearly, I thought, he never could sit still either. Mine were always recombed and snipped incrementally toward an impossible ideal. And Mommy's tireless precision nitpicking paid off during the kindergarten invasion of head lice.

"Your glorious hair," she would say, "like Rapunzel's, it makes you unique. Let ordinary girls wear it short. Ach! We don't give in to lice!"

As a young woman in Berlin during World War II, where she had met and enchanted my American soldier father, she had gained experience with lice in her periodic migrations to bomb shelters. Now she poured vinegar on my shafts with sneering expertise, while distracting me with exotic tales of the *Arabian Nights* and of Scheherazade. My hair, like a Persian rug, she said, was my own magic flying carpet. Adventures and romance would be mine. Taking care of my hair seemed part of the fare.

MY FOURTEENTH BIRTHDAY was memorable because of my hair. While I was on a court-ordered visit to Wisconsin, my estranged father gave me the last gift he was ever to give me:

an expensive boar-bristle hairbrush with a wooden handle. In the years to come, I would hand the hairbrush to whichever gangly suitor was seated with me on our love seat. It was tacitly a courtship audition and routine.

Though my mother was often away from home working, it's during this period that my most real, most cherished images of her reside, when she was already in her late forties and early fifties. In her youth, she had done some modeling and had gone to finishing school in Europe. Now her restored confidence and inner and outer beauty had returned. She wore her black hair piled, pinned, and tucked behind a long curtain of bangs. Her hair set off the red Avon lipstick she wore as well as sold. On top of her head, a coiled hairpiece was a unique engineering feat designed, she liked to say, to achieve "height." She braced it with a scaffold of U-shaped hairpins, anchored in the back with a curved comb: a banister that first raked and then cupped the upsweep. She built this tower every weekday morning and deconstructed it every night. In a cloud of Adorn hairspray, she tied a dimestore scarf under her chin, and in her thirdhand Volkswagen, off she putt-putt-putted to work. On weekends she wrapped her hair in one of her many hand-knit turbans, like a big swami-knot tiara, again, to conjure height.

One day shortly before I left home for college in New York, while my mother was at work, I shredded my hick yearbook photo: long hair in a tacky Clairol auburn rinse, a corn-fed early draft of "me." I made a rare phone call to my dad, to tell him my news—which I hadn't told him when it was news. The daughter he barely knew was calling to report that she had been accepted to Barnard College! Heart pounding, dry mouth, I sputtered out, "Hi . . . it's Debbie." "Debbie . . . who?" was his reply. My moment of sweet triumph was crushed, along with my invitation to make him proud of me. The conversation did not last much longer, but his question became my *quo vadis.*

*Debbie who?* Debbie who? Is it any wonder that for decades my hair became a living, tangible way for me to try to answer that question?

I set off from Peoria for New York City, fantasizing that my handsome father might come looking for me one day—which of course I hoped he would. If I had cut my hair, how would he recognize me? And how could I reject the one gift he gave me, that totemic hairbrush, which went to Barnard with me? It was a perfect all-in-one icon of unrequited love, of pain and pleasure. It was my dad magnet.

I spent the next several years in some sort of restless cycle, dating lovely guys and then breaking up with them abruptly, as I tried desperately to find some substitute for a father's sort of love.

Steadily I advanced in a career at the *New York Times*, one that I adored and that was a vessel large enough to contain this sense of myself as a heroine in my own jagged romantic tale. Well into my time there, I met Eric, the man I would marry, who loved to brush my hair with a boar-bristle hairbrush on the love seat in my apartment. My inner concubine had found her permanent sultan, and we found love together long and durable and magical. With him, I was able to authentically integrate all the parts of my being. And he loved me for them. When motherhood came, I was the long-haired, serene Madonna with child. In years to come, our toddler son played with my hair and my dear stepson gripped the strands while in my arms on the playground, as if for security. At night my husband stroked my hair tenderly.

As my mother aged, her neck muscles could not support her Erector set underpinnings to what were now silver wisps, her too-heavy metal sunk in a flimsy anchorage. She died in bed, at ninety-one, on Mother's Day, 2009, her twist of hair held in one small comb. Her final words surprised me, but they should not have. "Meine Debbieleine, you must try to keep your beautiful long hair out of your eyes . . ." Then off she putt-putted for good.

Her longevity gave me hope. I had expected for so long to die young of the congenital cardiomyopathy that had taken my brother, Peter, born on Pearl Harbor Day in 1948, who died at fifty-three on Labor Day, 2002, of this heart muscle weakness we inherited from Dad, who died at fifty-two, without our having reconciled.

It was under that burden of holiday superstition that

just before Labor Day in 2012, I shuffled toward our medicine cabinet, doubled over in abdominal pain. I pawed my sloppy hair and grabbed a butterfly claw to jerk it back. It was only by chance, bent over in pain, and with new eyeglasses, that I noticed that these tiny claws, which I had bought by the scoop from a Canal Street vendor, were etched with a "Hello Kitty." How lapsed, my vanity.

> *As my mother aged, her neck muscles could not support her Erector set underpinnings to what were now silver wisps, her too-heavy metal sunk in a flimsy anchorage.*

Eric insisted that I go to our doctor immediately. My agony won him his case. The doctor felt my abdomen and dispatched us urgently to the hospital, where tests confirmed that I had ovarian cancer, stage 3. When I heard the diagnosis pronounced, I flashed back ridiculously to that cartoon character, Snagglepuss, saying, "Exit . . . stage left!" This period would forever after be known by what our twenty-year-old son, Peter, called "Mom's incanceration."

Surgery just after Labor Day went smoothly, and my guts were stitched up dirndl-style. Realizing that once chemo began, my hair would shortly fall out in clumps, I soon decided that if I was going to "exit, stage 3," I was going to be badass and bald. Eric and I set off for Supercuts for a preemptive buzz. It was Eric's idea to get his own hair buzzed too, down to the scalp, in support. We treated it as a date, not doom. I had regressive moments. Sitting at the Supercuts on First Avenue at Sixty-Ninth Street, about to lose all my hair, I felt so deeply loved by my husband—the most loved I had ever felt in my life, by any man. In some enormous shift there at the budget hair franchise, he transformed himself into not only my husband but also the father and older brother I had lost too, all in one lovely, beaming bald man. Our photo, taken by the hair-cutter, is my favorite after our wedding photo. He tenderly stroked my bald head each night as he had always done when I had long hair. Every marriage should have an anniversary in which both go bald.

Then came months of chemotherapy. Each cycle began with drawing vials of blood. "Decanting," said our friend Kathleen. "It's the right term for the wife of a wine critic." With all the urgings to "drink this," "stand there," "swallow these" (fistfuls of steroids), and for all the sharp needle sticks and intubations, I thought my own name was Sit Still. Cancer and chemotherapy drew me into a disempowering undertow that made me feel like a child again. Decisions about hair were once again freighted with control issues.

I wanted no wig. Scarves appeared, though not dime-store ones like Mom's. Friends presented hand-knit cashmere berets, cotton prints from Provence, Hermès silken twill and street-vendor beanies, bandannas, and a gendarme kepi. I raked my haul toward me like chips, a VIP high roller at

Cancer Casino Royale. Who knew that chemo was truly the big grift?

Soon, though, it became a burden to put visitors at ease with my baldness or to show I appreciated their gifts. I had also begun to embrace baldness. And one day in the shower, I felt water pooling around my ankles. I shrieked and looked down, feeling an absurd relief to see that the mass at the drain was my own body hair, not the dead mouse I had imagined. No more shaving under my arms and my legs. Downy forearm hair was gone too. Flecks in the toilet water: those were an armada of pubic hair sailing away. By my son's birthday, which is Halloween, I was Mrs. Potato Head dispensing treats. With neither eyebrows nor eyelashes, my irises were red from debris.

I learned that some cancer patients adopt a pet to caress. I turned to knitting. In my twenties, I had designed complex Aran cable patterns. Now, my brain—a filthy sponge soaked with rat poisons—was a slurry of compromised memory, double vision, diminished dexterity and focus. I could not remember even beginner stitch sequences. Nonetheless, I pushed through and bought supplies online. Exotic yarns arrived in sync with hopped-up steroid cycles. I could not die as long as there were long, braided skeins of alpaca and yak, merino and cashmere, in hair shades: timber, hazelnut, bruin, wolf, birch, to satisfy the mournful longing to handle my own. I was like a little girl once more, waiting for my mother to braid my hair, each new thick hank of yarn demanding that I wind it. I could still know pleasure, and forget my situation and even the close breath of death, for a while, through these plaits. And each wound bun reminded me of my mom. Boomerang-shaped cable-stitch hooks were metaphorical hairpins.

After the first chemo, I struggled to detangle any knot in the wool. The first time, I stuck it out for three hours, pretending I was removing chewing gum from a child's hair. I would not use scissors. I was like Mom with her lice management. Neuropathy, a painful and numbing side effect of chemo, sometimes permanent if not countered with activity, drove me to set a pace of maniacal productivity as occupational therapy. Knitting silk appeased the twitches. As vertigo and spastic kicking rendered me more sedentary, I knitted much as I had once tended my dolls' hair, stooped in introspection.

My family nickname is Hedgie, for "hedgehog": prickly, reclusive, and so misunderstood. By February of 2013, I was in remission. I looked and felt that nickname. By Mother's Day, soft, downy hair emerged, and I had a chic boyish look. By mid-July, tight Persian-lamb curls capered close to the scalp. By summer's end, I was finger-twirling Little Debbie snack-cake waves.

When friends asked what my plan was for my hair, I was defensive. I deflected them obliquely, while within I nursed a maternal protectiveness, inchoate yet absolute, as if they were intrusively asking about my child. It was at that time in my office that I had casually begun to reach for a binder clip to keep my hair back, or better, a tiny green florist clamp off my orchid stem.

The following Thanksgiving, my hair had returned, but I was frowsy, dishing up brussels sprouts like a matronly Edith Bunker. Stubbornly, I resisted grooming what felt like my hair's reassertion of itself. I mothered the mop, which now flopped over my ears haphazardly. I alone could understand this precocious hair, entitled as it was to run amok. To cut and style it would be to banish a spirited girl for running indoors; I yearned to see what this hair sought to do on its own. And, I confess, fussing with my hair meant surrendering the saintly pedestal of the illness, the prolonged privileges and considerations I earned as Miss Cancer. This messy hair was a halo that conferred spiritual superiority and martyrdom, as much as it was an affirmation that I was going to live. To alter its natural course would be presumptuous, greedy, like daring death by taking in stride an optimistic diagnosis. To groom it, I argued, would be like investing in a gamble and jinxing a scenario in which I was going to live.

*I confess, fussing with my hair meant surrendering the saintly pedestal of the illness, the prolonged privileges and considerations I earned as Miss Cancer.*

Right about then, something shifted inside me. Perhaps it was triggered by the ever more ludicrous attempts to carry off this mess on top. When I pocketed a long barrette-style bread-bag clamp from home, to keep my bangs out of my eyes, I thought of those troll dolls of my youth, whose rough hanks of dull hair I had coated in fragrant Alberto VO5 lanolin and clipped with small, colorful plastic tags from grocery bread-loaf bags. It was time. The movie persona of Gilda, played by Rita Hayworth—which I had adopted in undergraduate seductions at V and T Pizza in Morningside Heights—was in my distant past. I was no longer a smoldering inner stripper, her hair flouncing saucily as she crooned lyrically, "Put the blame on Mame." No, I had begun looking like Mamie Eisenhower.

After work on Christmas Eve, I slipped into Supercuts, the same branch where Eric and I had gotten our heads shaved. A stylist was preparing to close, but she invited me in. Silently, she snipped, she paused, sought my approval of her tidy trim through nods "yes" or shakes "no" to my mirrored reflection. It was done.

And now, more than a year later, I'm fifty-eight, with a new wavy, short but natural, groomed look.

What made my soft hair resurge was not merely the cessation of toxin, but its antidote, undiluted infusions of love from unexpected reservoirs. The hair coiled, groomed by fingers of invisible handlers, dead and living. These soft tufts are fresh and well-tended sod growing atop the shallow grave where my memories of cancer lie buried. I place photos of my unflattering transitional looks on my shelves alongside the ones of the child, the vamp, the adventurer, the dignified silhouette of a cameo, the Madonna and child. Like me, these waves are now gentler, more yielding. Eyelashes flirt, brows arch. There are no bad-hair days. I continue to knit bouncy ribbed scarves. Their juicy stretch and gauge replicate Mom's fortune-teller turbans. When I can no longer pin my hair, these will probably wrap my head too. After all, as my mother taught me, a girl sometimes needs some height.

# At Last, I Learn
# How to Turn Heads

. . . . . . . . . . . . . . . . . . . . . . . . . . . . . . . . . . . . . . . .

JANE SMILEY

**S**everal years ago, and unexpectedly, I admit, my beauty regimen of what my family would call "utter neglect" but I prefer to term "halfhearted efforts" for once paid off. I was in Edinburgh. It was early in the morning. I put on a bit of lipstick (Guerlain Terracotta) that I had gotten in a duty-free shop and I looked in the mirror and said, "Wow." I looked fabulous. I turned my head. I still looked fabulous. I smiled. I looked even better. I looked so great that I didn't even mind that there was no one to see me. The proximate cause of my wonderful, heart-stopping, and unprecedented hotness was a haircut and color I'd gotten before leaving the States. What happened was, I had gotten to the San Francisco airport after a two-hour drive up US 101 only to realize while standing in the Air France line that

I had left my passport in another handbag (which was neatly put away back home in Carmel Valley).

I then tried to impose myself on my sister in Palo Alto for the evening, but she and her husband had a romantic date and didn't seem to want to invite me along. So I ambled down University Avenue, with a big rubber band from an accordion folder keeping my hair out of my face, and I saw a salon. After long consideration, I decided to go in and have my hair done and my eyebrows waxed (you can't really see my eyebrows because of my glasses, but I like that feeling when the wax and hair are stripped away—it wakes you right up).

My stylist was efficient and had a nice haircut herself, but I couldn't see what she was doing without my glasses. All I knew was, the hairstyle that I chose from the styling book was called Femme Fatale. Or maybe it was Harlot. Uncombed and a little tangled, it was distinct from all the others in the book. The color my stylist came up with had not really ever been seen on a natural-born human before, but it was a great color. My head looked like it had been gold-plated, a happy color, not an authentic color, and that was good too. I am way too old to be trying to fake it. The

*All I knew was, the hairstyle that I chose from the styling book was called Femme Fatale. Or maybe it was Harlot.*

bonus I got with this haircut was that I could put a hat on, take it off, and have the hair fly out to its intended shape again. It was just like Barbie in every way.

*The bonus I got with this haircut was that I could put a hat on, take it off, and have the hair fly out to its intended shape again. It was just like Barbie in every way.*

And the eyebrows! One of the features of the salon was that the music and the chitchat were so loud that I could neither make myself heard nor intelligently answer questions, so whenever they asked me what I wanted, I just smiled and nodded. In this—as in all things—it is better to leave it to the experts, and the eyebrow lady was an expert.

As soon as I became a beauty, I came up with some tips, which I will now share.

1. Try to look your best as infrequently as possible. However you look, people get used to it. If you accustom them to a very high standard—your hair and makeup are always perfect, your clothing is expensive and fetching—you are just setting them up for disappointment if you make a mistake or, God forbid, get lazy. If, however, you do as I do and wear jeans and a T-shirt most of the time and wear makeup only for special occasions, there is always the possibility of a pleasant surprise. No, they didn't know you had any taste. No, it was not clear

that you were actually pretty, but you are! This is not the same as letting yourself go. It is more like being dormant, so that from time to well-chosen time you may blossom.

2.  Never make shopping an event. The job of a flattering outfit is to improve itself upon you. If you need or want something for a particular event, you will certainly buy something you don't like. It's much better, for example, to take your son to the mall and run into your favorite store, grab something that strikes you off the rack, run into the dressing room, decide right then and there, and leave as soon as it is paid for to make sure your son doesn't hog the video-game demo at the game store. When you look for something, you will buy it; when you don't look for something, you will love it.

3.  Go blond when you go gray. Dark hair is for children. It goes nicely with smooth, creamy skin. Once your mane is striped and your face is lined, there are too many contrasts. You look too complicated. Nice color highlights look like an optical illusion and are a good way to start. Think tawny.

4.  Kiss a lot. For whatever reason, usually a bad one based on habits of disapproval and self-righteousness, the lips of middle-aged women thin out and eventually disappear. The best antidote to this is kissing every day for extended periods of time. Your partner should really put his (or her) heart

into this—the tendency of your lips to disappear needs to be aggressively counteracted. You need to soften your lips so that they can be worked with effectively.

After I became a beauty, I experienced something that, I suspect, all beauties experience. My surface, head to toe, took on a life of its own. People reacted to it. I reacted to it, but not as though it were me. More as though it were a separate being, a Tall Blond, rather remote, but with a knowing look in her eye. It almost didn't matter what she did; she got away with anything. People smiled at her. Men looked at her—first at the hair, then at the other parts. Almost inevitably, because I am over six feet tall, there was some speculation about her. Was she a woman? Was she a female impersonator? She had just that hint of ambiguity that draws the gaze. This had happened to me before, but when I had short, dark hair, the way it worked was that guys would say, "Hey, buddy, you need something?" and I would answer in my regular female voice, and they would do a double take and get embarrassed and start calling me "ma'am." For years, I was tall but unobvious, rather like a tree. For a month or two, several years ago, there she was, the beauty. I was with her. I suspect it's this way for most beauties.

After I had been a beauty for a while, I began to think, So what?My life is what it is, and I like it. I began to wonder what being a beauty is for, after all. Beauty in women is usually seen as a negotiable commodity with some value in the marriage market, or as an add-on to another, more specialized talent. In our media culture, beauty is likely to be a good thing because it might be parlayed into bucks. At any rate, though, beauty is restless—it promises that anything can happen.

But I didn't want anything to happen. My partner thought I was beautiful already, my kids didn't care, and my friends didn't notice. And the entire literary history of beauty is marked by suspicion and regret. A poet can't look at a beautiful girl without seeing the skull within the skin or, at least, the old harridan within the youthful darling. Total hotness, as Shakespeare said, "hath all too short a date."

Or does it? In that month or two, one thing I noticed was that there was a great deal of beauty around me. Not only the usual things—like horses, valley mists, blown roses dropping petals—but also sudden, striking sights: lush grass that seemed to be giving off a green light; a restaurant in Paris entirely walled in Art Nouveau mirrors; a woman with magenta hair, lips like a purple bow, and freckles that looked like polka dots (trust me—she was astonishing); an old friend who looked stooped and subdued when I saw her three years ago, around the time of her divorce, but who now looked active and free (and just my age! Do we constitute a statistical sample?); and of course men, women, and children of all sorts, all ages (mostly young, though, I admit). Shakespeare's line was wrong, I think. The drive to see beauty and to be beautiful is a permanent feature of human nature. Beauty is fleeting when we try to capture or possess it, even when we declare that we have located it in a particular loved one, but it is constant and unchanging when we only watch it come and go, like time itself.

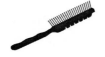

# Getting Real

· · · · · · · · · · · · · · · · · · · · · · · · · · · · · · · · · · · · · · · · · · · · · · · · · · ·

ANNE KREAMER

I began consciously playing with my identity in 1964, when Louise Fitzhugh published *Harriet the Spy*. I was a highly regimented nine-year-old Catholic convent-school girl, and the quirky, free-spirited Harriet became my heroine. She solved mysteries. She was *interesting*. I mimicked everything she did. I carried a notebook in which I scrawled observations—as I skulked around neighbors' houses trying to see if anything was out of the ordinary, threatening to share with my parents my older sister's habit of putting on forbidden stockings after she left the house on her way to meet her friends and the neighborhood boys. Regrettably, nothing very captivating happened on my Kansas City block.

In 1968, as I turned thirteen, Julie Barnes, the character

played by Peggy Lipton in the groovy crime series *The Mod Squad,* abruptly usurped Harriet as the person I wanted to emulate. Her character amped up Harriet's domestic spying by orders of magnitude. Julie was an *undercover* cop. She had a black partner. She was a hippie with straight, long blond hair. She seemed effortlessly chic (not that I really grasped that concept at thirteen) in her jeans and leather jackets. The show's urban grit, drugs, and antiwar imagery were beyond any imitation available in my thoroughly *Leave It to Beaver* 1960s suburban teen world—but Peggy's hair, *that* I could do. I could grow my chin-length blond hair long, hoping that groovier hair would make me as fascinating as she seemed. Growing my hair at thirteen was the gateway drug for what became a lifelong practice of using a change in my hair as a way to achieve a shift in my sense of self.

With the enthusiasm of extreme youth, I failed at first to appreciate that long hair was not something that could be achieved quickly. Hair grows at the speed hair grows, which is slowly—on average, about half an inch a month. It took *forever* in teen time—the entirety of my high school years and *Mod Squad*'s existence—for my hair to finally reach my waist. But even before it was actually long, *consciously* deciding for the first time how I wanted to look made me feel grown up in an adult kind of way.

I held on to that agency when I decided to reinvent myself before leaving for college. I pulled that hard-earned mane

into a ponytail, and in one snip, I ruthlessly cut it all off. *Bam!*
In a few seconds, I was a new person. At least in my own
mind. I was no longer the long-haired teenager, no siree, I
was now a not-quite-Twiggy ingenue. During the next four
years, changes to my hair took a backseat to more dramatic
sex-drugs-and-rock-and-roll identity explorations. But when I
entered the workforce, I once again began to experiment with
different hair-based personae. An early job in banking was the
catalyst for the first time I dyed my hair a dramatic color—the
wholly unnatural-looking, bittersweet orange that the fashion designer Vivienne Westwood has made her trademark. I
wanted to make very clear that I was a *bohemian*, not some
beigy banker type.

Later, when I worked in television and publishing, I didn't
need to use such an obviously artificial color to assert my artsy
bona fides, and I softened the harsh orange into a warmer rus-
set. At forty, panicking about middle age, I once again turned
to a new hair color as a coping mechanism, dyeing my hair
black, intending to project a Joan Jettish, I'm-not-old-I'm-
a-rocker kind of vibe. It was a disastrous failure. "You look
like your evil twin," a friend of mine actually said. Both of my
daughters, who were then five and seven, burst into tears the
evening I came home with the new color. I had to live with that
mistake for a long time, because you cannot simply wash ebony
dye out of naturally light brownish hair, any more than you can
grow your hair down to your waist in a hurry. Chastened by my

hasty decision, once the black faded and grew out, I settled into a uniform mahogany shade.

Sometime in my midforties, I noticed a dramatic shift in my relationship with time, as processed through the growth of my hair. Instead of the half inch of growth every month marking how slowly time seemed to pass, the opposite happened. Time sped up. To maintain the "natural" brown hue, I had to color my hair every six weeks, every five, every four, and finally every three weeks to keep the gray from showing. It wasn't that my hair was growing in faster, of course, but that as more gray grew in, the contrast between dye and roots became much more pronounced.

The speed at which the roots seemed to grow yanked me out of the here and now, and I began to obsess over the near future, measuring life moment to moment through the template of how many days a month my hair would look good. By this time, my hair-looking-good window was mercilessly short—four or five days between when the smudge of dye had faded from my temples and hairline and when the roots started coming in. Part of my decision to quit dyeing my hair at forty-seven was a desire to liberate myself from that relentless clock. The other catalyst was my looking at a photograph of myself standing between my then sixteen-year-old butter-blond daughter and a dear gray-haired friend. Sandwiched between those two naturally colored heads of hair, I thought my helmet of dark brown dye looked terrible.

I had a visceral reaction. I hated it. It was that simple. The color had to go.

I'd anticipated that eliminating the five hours a month I spent on the salon commute and sitting in a colorist's chair would make my weeks feel more expansive. I was right about that. I discovered that the average American woman spends even more time than I had on professional hair maintenance at the salon—a staggering 7.9 hours a month, or the equivalent of *two* full-time workweeks a year. But most of us never quantify these hours—I surely hadn't—because it would force an uncomfortable awareness of the opportunity cost of how those hours (and thousands of dollars) might have been better spent.

Knowing from my ebony fiasco that there is no easy way to get rid of hair dye, and fearing the loss of my resolve, I offered to write a diary of the experience for *More* magazine. I was right to build in that layer of accountability. I had to work with my colorist, first adding blondish highlights to blend into the gray, trying to mask the ice floe shelf of gray that was glacially creeping down my head. It was six months into the process before I quit dyeing altogether. The reader response to my *More* piece was so overwhelming that I decided to dig deeper, eventually publishing a book, *Going Gray: What I Learned about Beauty, Sex, Work, Motherhood, Authenticity, and Everything Else That Really Matters.*

I'd fretted that having gray hair would make me feel even more invisible than a middle-aged woman ordinarily feels.

But I was happily shocked to discover the opposite. Until I had my own unique scattershot blend of gray, steel, buck-

*I'd fretted that having gray hair would make me feel even more invisible than a middle-aged woman ordinarily feels. But I was happily shocked to discover the opposite.*

wheat, white, and pearl strands of hair, I'd been blind to the fact that I was merely one of a million women sporting *exactly* the same hair-color-industrial-complex shade of "rich medium neutral brown." Does any word connote invisibility more than *neutral*? I could see now that, rather than making me look young and vibrant, my color had had the unintended consequence of commodifying me, making me part of an army of "rich medium neutral browns." Without dye, I was learning that the singular, complex hybrid tone created by the various natural colors on my scalp allowed me, for the first time, to genuinely individuate myself. I'd accidentally discovered something the psychologist Daniel Gilbert writes about in *Stumbling on Happiness*, that blending in with the masses denies us one of the key drivers we have for happiness—celebrating our uniqueness. I promise you, no one else has my particular shade of gray. And I'm often the only woman in the room with hair that's not dyed.

Much to my surprise, when I stopped coloring my hair,

time began to slow down, in a good way. That the process takes a while, not subject to any instant fix, turned out this time around to be a gift. It took eighteen long months (including a radically short cut) for the color to completely grow out. I came to understand, as I said in my book, that "in some ways letting my hair go gray was a bit like an intensive five-day-a-week-on-the-therapist's-couch crash course, but with no shrink to guide me."

Allowing my gray hair to grow in, without going to the effort of hiding it, required me to give up the fantasy that I'd had the power to freeze my age to that time before I went gray. It forced me to confront my half-conscious fears about aging every time I looked in the mirror. The slow journey allowed me the time to process the fact that I now have less time ahead of me than I do behind me. This brought to mind the cultural historian Arden Reed's study of what he calls "slow art" and the work of the Long Now Foundation, cofounded by the musician Brian Eno and the creator of the *Whole Earth Catalogue*, Stewart Brand. "Civilization," Brand wrote in his Long Now manifesto, "is revving itself into a pathologi-

*Much to my surprise, when I stopped coloring my hair, time began to slow down, in a good way.*

cally short attention span. The trend might be coming from the acceleration of technology, the short-horizon perspective of market-driven economics, the next-election perspective of democracies, or the distractions of personal multi-tasking. All are on the increase. Some sort of balancing corrective to the short-sightedness is needed—some mechanism or myth which encourages the long view and the taking of long-term responsibility." Removing the illusory camouflage of hair dye grabbed me by the roots (pun intended) and forced me to take a longer view, to meditate on the passing of time in real time.

Rather than depressing me, every glance in the mirror at my gray hair has become a carpe diem moment. Artificial hair color no longer lulls me into a false sense of security—or, rather, quasi obliviousness—about the passage of time, the inevitability of death. And this, it turns out, is healthy—and it has raised my spirits. In her 1993 study of aging, *The Fountain of Age*, Betty Friedan wrote that "an accurate, realistic, active identification with one's own aging—as opposed both to resignation to the stereotype of being 'old' and denial of age changes—seems an important key to vital aging, and even longevity . . . . [I]t takes a conscious breaking out of youthful definitions—for man or woman—to free oneself for continued development in age."

*Rather than depressing me, every glance in the mirror at my gray hair has become a carpe diem moment.*

I've earned my grays. As I enter the phase of life when

illness begins more and more to strike down friends and family, I become more and more grateful for the simple gift of being alive. As I approach my seventh decade, I want to slow time down. A decade ago, when I stopped dyeing, I had no idea that watching the ways my pewter and gunmetal strands of hair have morphed over time into pearls and silvers would help me do that. The naturalist Akiko Busch writes of something called the ecotone, which is the zone where two habitats merge, "that threshold where water meets the shore, where the forest comes to meadow, or where woodland ends at a cultivated lawn." She suggests that it is in "the intensity and complexity in these places of transition, where one thing manages to become another," that we are fully aware of the possibilities of change. The *very* gradual but ever-present transition of my hair color into white is my personal ecotone. Keen observation of the incremental changes in my natural hair color keeps me alert to the passage of time, of the need to *live now*. My hair and I are finally in equilibrium with time—the days and years are neither hurtling past nor artificially stationary. My hair is now like the second hand on life's clock, keeping me right where I need to be.

# No, I Won't Go Gray

. . . . . . . . . . . . . . . . . . . . . . . . . . . . . . . . . . . . . . . . . . . . . . . . . . . . . . . .

## ELIZABETH BENEDICT

I have never gotten high marks in fashion and beauty. If I had to grade myself, I'd say I usually hover around a B-. On special occasions, I can sometimes work my way up to an A-. If I got a report card from the universe—or maybe from my sister—I'm sure it would say, Liz's appearance would probably improve if she could see her way clear to a better attitude.

It's what comes, I think, of working at home in my pajamas for so many decades; of having come of age in the time of Joan Baez at the Newport Folk Festival and Indian bedspreads as fashion statements; of having a social life that rarely requires a dress; and of always having other matters I preferred to obsess over—sentences, paragraphs, paintings, who is president, how I would pay my health insurance premiums, and the state of my love life.

I have gone to plenty of posh places in my time and cobbled together whatever I needed to wear—the specifics of which escape me now—but the only event for which I ever put on a long, even quasi-formal dress was my sister's wedding ten years ago. The bridesmaids had been instructed to wear black dresses of our choosing; if I wore pants, as I preferred, my sister said I could not be a bridesmaid. I had never been a bridesmaid (my friends tend to marry at nonweddings, like my own, at city halls or Buddhist temples in countries so far away not even family members are expected to come), but I didn't want to be quite so sidelined at this event. I overcame my resistance and found a narrow Ann Taylor crepe-textured dress at my favorite thrift store and wore it without incident, although I felt a bit out of sorts dressed up as a girly girl.

Days later, when a family friend who hadn't been there said to me, "My mother saw you at the wedding and said you looked fabulous," I cringed. I know it was a perverse response. Isn't that the point of going out, of getting "dressed up"—that people will notice and approve? Why couldn't I embrace "fabulous" when the alternative is whatever the opposite of that is—ordinary, forgettable, neutral, meh? What's this all about?

There is something about the tyranny of what is expected of women that I resist, that makes me want to reject the pressure, the feelings of being on display and of being judged. There seems to me a kind of desperation in the desire to be ornamental, to be *too* put together, too pleasing, too slavish to the demands of fashion. "Although they do not talk of it at school," W. B. Yeats tells us in "Adam's Curse," women must "labour to be beautiful," and I read the lines, enjoying the lovely rhyme (school/beautiful), but then I think, Still? Haven't we learned anything in a hundred years? (Answer: yes, Botox, Restylane, and face-lifts.) And there's this: there are so many women who are better at this than I am (my sister, for one), who actually enjoy doing whatever needs to be done to look a whole lot spiffier than I look, that I'm happy just to sit this activity out, like the klutz who has the good sense to avoid the dance floor.

I'm plenty comfortable displaying the words I write, and the ideas and characters I make public, but when it comes to calling attention to my clothes, I would rather wear the writer's equivalent of a little black dress and pearls, which is to say, something plain but not nearly that fancy. Reading a fashion magazine recently at a doctor's office, I learned about Roberta Armani, niece of Giorgio, who helps run the family business. She said of her own wardrobe, "I try to be present but not ostentatious." At last, I thought, a kindred spirit!—never mind that we're present at vastly different places, she at Paris Fashion Week and I at the Salvation Army thrift store in Hell's Kitchen.

Yet I am not oblivious to the seductions of fashion or the

allure of the beautiful. I look often at art and try to surround myself with as much of it as possible. When I gape at pictures of Michelle Obama's otherworldly wardrobe—which I do compulsively—I ask myself, What would *I* wear to state dinners if *my* husband were president? Would I dare to wear Narciso Rodriguez, or would I bore the world to death with my Eileen Fisher hand-me-downs accentuated with a purple scarf and silver stud earrings?

Which brings me, of course, to my hair, and it's here where my shtick about not caring much about my appearance gives way to a boatload of vanity. The older I get, it seems, the more attention I pay to my hair, and the more outright fakery I'm willing to bankroll and endure. Little Miss "I Can't Be Bothered" is not quite a lioness protecting her cubs, but faced with a scalp full of gray roots, the last thing I intend to do is let nature take her course. It was not always the case.

When I was a young teenager, in the thrall of Ms. Baez, my dark hair, like hers, hung down my back for years that stretched into decades. Mine was thick, a little wavy, and frizzy on humid days. If only, I think now, I had had a flat-iron, I would have saved my mother having to iron my locks on the ironing board. That phase didn't go on for long, though I can't say how many such treatments I demanded. Floating around somewhere in my memory are some big pink plastic rollers and some Dippity-do that I know I used to smooth out my hair, but for how long or when, pre- or post-ironing-board, I have no clue. My hair wasn't curly in an interesting way, but nor was it frizzy in a way that made me want to shoot myself.

Perhaps if it had been more extreme—more extremely distressing—I would have vivid memories of the solutions I had sought. But back then, I'm not sure solutions existed, aside from those giant rollers. "Going to the beauty parlor," which my mother did every week to groom her short, once very red hair, was about sitting under a gigantic heating bubble for half an hour, until the hair baked around a collection of rollers smashed against the scalp. The hair was then

*The older I get, it seems, the more attention I pay to my hair, and the more outright fakery I'm willing to bankroll and endure.*

brushed, smoothed, and sprayed to a helmet-like glaze—the poor woman's Jackie Kennedy bouffant.

I don't remember when handheld dryers came into my life, nor when blow-drying hair to make it sleek and smooth did either, but it was long after Joan Baez finished singing "Sad-Eyed Lady of the Lowlands." I can't remember getting my hair cut once in college and only recall a single visit to a cheap salon in my late twenties, for what must have been a trim. Around that time, I belonged to a gym where I swam regularly and loved drying my hair there, with the boxy wall-mounted dryer in the locker room, so I could pull, brush, and straighten the hair with two hands and thereby make it smoother than I could if I had to hold a dryer with one hand. This must have been the beginning of some spark of hair vanity. I also have vague memories of buying packets of special conditioner, because of the beating the chlorine gave my hair. Were those ninety-nine-cent packets what is called "product"? I have no idea. I was absent when discussions about "product" began—and only recently learned that the singular is the accepted form of the word. Why not "products"? I still don't get it.

*I can't bear admitting to myself that I belong to a cult, albeit millions of members strong, whose core belief— whose only belief—is that our fake hair color is essential to our well-being.*

When I quit my job to write my first novel—and was no longer in the vicinity of that gym and those dreamy wall dryers—I thought I might never again find such a compatible way to do my hair. At that point, it never occurred to me that I would one day spend money, and fairly regularly, *getting my hair done. Going to the beauty parlor. Dying it,* for heaven's sake, doing exactly what my mother did before Betty Friedan and Gloria Steinem changed the game and told us we did not have to be Playboy Bunnies or baby dolls or arm candy anymore. We could go natural, we could examine our cervixes for fun and otherwise just *be ourselves.*

It still seems ridiculous to me when I'm in the midst of it, sitting in a room with dozens of women soaking our heads in toxic chemicals, paying hundreds of dollars—just that week—to pretend to look like people we are not. I can't bear admitting to myself that I belong to a cult, albeit millions of members strong, whose core belief—whose only belief—is that our fake hair color is essential to our well-being. But it does *seem* to be the case that the fake color, the ABG (anything but gray), *is* essential to our sanity, as are the blow-dryer, the flat-iron, the hot combs, the chemical relaxers, the thousand-dollar hair weaves—the whole multibazillion-dollar hair industry.

A year ago, I met a stylish, sophisticated woman—Anne Kreamer—who had gone gray and written a book about it and informally advises those who want to take that treacherous journey. She told me how I could make the lengthy transition and said that because I had short hair—yes, I'd long ago lopped off my teenage tresses—it would be fairly easy. Although I think about it *every* time I look in the mirror and notice the gray roots beneath the warm brown that used to be authentically mine, I balk. No, I think, not now, not yet. I'm embarrassed by my vanity, but I'd be more embarrassed to go gray, gracefully or any other way.

I come up with all kinds of excuses for why I keep signing up for Superficiality, Inauthenticity, Fake Hair, the Big Con. Reason 1: I work with high school and college students, and if I look like I'm their grandmother, they will not pay attention to what I'm saying. (Note to self: Their grandmothers probably don't have gray hair. They might never have seen gray hair on women!) Reason 2: If I go gray and it looks awful, then going back to brown will be even more embarrassing than never having left it. Reason 3: The going-gray guru, who offered to help me, looks fabulous, but I'm certain I'll never look half as good (see reason 2). Reason 4: Given the modest state of my wardrobe, I need all the help I can get. Why not go to town when it comes to my hair?

*I'm embarrassed by my vanity, but I'd be more embarrassed to go gray, gracefully or any other way.*

But the real reasons I'm not budging are the most pressing, the most fundamental: I don't want to be reminded of my age. I don't want anyone else to be reminded of it. I want to continue to pretend for as long as I can, as long as the money holds out, and the energy to keep up the charade. There may come a day when that changes, but in the meantime, I'm still with Ponce de León in Florida, in search of the Fountain of Youth.

Speaking of Florida. Speaking of the Fountain of Youth. On a recent visit to Miami Beach, I was delighted that the apartment I'd rented was near a branch of the Beauty Schools of America, where a sign on the door welcomes walk-in customers to be worked on by students. I was growing my hair out at the time—I wanted only a blow-dry, not a cut or color—and the price was ten dollars. Ten dollars! It was fine that the student didn't speak English, and fine that she took more than an hour to dry my hair. When I got back to the apartment, I took a bunch of selfies because I thought my hair looked terrific. Really terrific. Especially for ten bucks. Four days later, I went back for another blow-dry. This time the stylist was faster, spoke English, and had a sweet, serious personality. Her name was Sahara. She took only forty-five minutes, and again, my hair looked great. I was over the moon.

When I went to pay, I told the woman at the desk what I had had done. "Five dollars," she said.

"But it was ten dollars last week."

"It's the Tuesday discount," she said. "Five dollars if you're a senior."

"A senior! I'm not a senior. How could you think I'm a senior?"

"Because it's Tuesday. All the seniors come on Tuesdays."

I dropped a ten-dollar bill on the counter and sprinted out of the place, churning excuses for how this could have happened—that I'd been mistaken for an old lady. She was a kid herself, I reasoned, so everyone looks old. She barely looked at me, I reasoned, so how could she accurately assess my age? And on and on I ranted to myself, winning and then losing debating points, and remembering what the going-gray guru had told me a year ago: "Even with hair color, no one thinks you're a kid."

DENIAL IS A powerful drug. Ponce de León was onto something. I returned to New York a short time later in search, not of the gray guru—her counseling services would have to wait—but of another cut-rate beauty salon where I could continue to indulge my demented fantasies. For several years, I'd been going irregularly to the Aveda salon in my neighborhood, where I requested the stylists and colorists in training, because their rates were lower than the pros. But even with those discounts, it's a pricey place, and I'd worked out a system where I'd get color one month and a haircut the next, which meant that I looked sort of OK—now and then. Present, you might say, but not ostentatious.

I had recently moved a few blocks and kept passing by a salon whose prices in the window were a fraction of Aveda's. One evening I walked in and took the first stylist who was available. Before long, I felt I was on the set of the beloved though short-lived British TV series *Fawlty Towers*, in which John Cleese plays the owner of a hotel-restaurant where disasters appear as often as dust mites. My stylist stopped doing my hair to yell at her colleagues. They yelled back. My stylist stormed off to berate the receptionist. She took it. The stylist confided in me, looking for an ally. "You have to come in every day to protect me," she said, in the way of a certain kind of crazy person. Again, she slipped away to give another stylist a piece of her mind. Everyone was furious. "We have customers here!" one of them shouted. This had the feeling of a familiar routine.

Chill, I kept saying to myself, this is seventy-five dollars, not a hundred and sixty. When it was all over, I looked pretty good. I was happy, hairwise, and what's wrong with a little drama? Perhaps this too is part of the whole laboring to be beautiful thing. I can take it. I really can.

When I get home, I decide to check in with another hair guru. Google assures me in hundreds of photos that Joan Baez is still looking good—but now she has a short, styled, wispy gray cut, close to the scalp. In truth, she looks fabulous. In the hundreds of photos I scan, she is gray and gorgeous. Should I? Shouldn't I? Yes. No. Maybe. Not now. Not yet. Maybe never. Maybe soon. The answer, my friend, just might be blowing in the wind.

# Contributors

**Elizabeth Benedict** is a graduate of Barnard College and the author of five novels, including the National Book Award finalist *Slow Dancing* and the best seller *Almost*, chosen as a top novel of the year 2001 by *Newsweek* and *Fresh Air*. She has edited two previous anthologies, the *New York Times* best seller *What My Mother Gave Me: Thirty-one Women on the Gifts That Mattered Most* (Algonquin) and *Mentors, Muses & Monsters: 30 Writers on the People Who Changed Their Lives*. She is the author of a book on writing fiction that's widely used in MFA programs, *The Joy of Writing Sex: A Guide for Fiction Writers*, and has published fiction and nonfiction in publications around the world, from the *New York Times* to *Daedalus* and Japanese *Playboy*. She's taught writing at Princeton, MIT, Swarthmore, and the Iowa Writers' Workshop and now coaches writers and edits manuscripts. She lives in New York City.

**Hallie Ephron** writes suspense novels she hopes readers won't be able to put down. Her work has been called "Hitchcockian" by *USA Today* and "deliciously creepy" by *Publishers Weekly*. Her award-winning best seller *Never Tell a Lie* was made into a movie for the Lifetime Movie Network. Her recent suspense novel *Night Night, Sleep Tight* (March 2015) takes readers back to early sixties Beverly Hills on waves of Aqua Net. She wrote a multi-award-nominated how-to book on mystery writing, *Writing and Selling Your Mystery Novel: How to Knock 'Em Dead with Style*, and teaches at writing conferences across the country. Hallie graduated from Barnard College and lives near Boston with her husband. She has two daughters and a granddaughter who can already catch and throw and run like the wind.

**Deborah Feldman** was born and raised in the Hasidic community of Satmar in Williamsburg, Brooklyn. She entered an arranged marriage at the age of seventeen, and her son was born two years later. At the age of twenty-five she published the *New York Times* best-selling memoir *Unorthodox: The Scandalous Rejection of My Hasidic Roots* (Simon and Schuster, 2012), and two years later she followed up with *Exodus*, a memoir of postreligious alienation and identity (Blue Rider Press, 2014.) Her essays have been published in the *Guardian*

*Observer, The Daily,* and *Salon,* as well as on CNN.com and Thirteen.org. Currently she is working on several new projects, including a novel and a documentary film, and is, most importantly, raising an amazing kid.

**Julia Fierro**'s debut novel,*Cutting Teeth,* was released by St. Martin's Press in 2014. Her work has been published in *Guernica, Poets & Writers, Glamour,* and other publications, and she has been profiled in the *L Magazine,* the *Observer,* and the *Economist.* In 2002, Julia founded the Sackett Street Writers' Workshop, and what started as eight writers meeting in her Brooklyn kitchen has grown into a creative home for over 2,500 writers. She is a graduate of the Iowa Writers' Workshop, where she was a Teaching-Writing Fellow, and currently teaches the post-MFA workshops at Sackett Street. Julia lives in Brooklyn with her husband and two children.

**Ru Freeman** is a Sri Lankan–born speaker, activist, and writer whose work has appeared internationally. She is the author of the novels *A Disobedient Girl* (2009) and *On Sal Mal Lane* (2013), both of which have been translated into multiple languages. She blogs for the *Huffington Post* on literature and politics.

**Myra Goldberg** is the author of *Whistling,* a book of stories, which was a *New York Times* Notable Book of the Year. Her novel, *Rosalind: A Family Romance,* was first published in *Representations of Motherhood* (Yale University Press). Her essays and stories have been published in magazines and anthologies in the United States, the UK, France, and Holland. She is finishing a book on storytelling and alternative families called *As It Turned Out* for Fordham University Press. She teaches writing at Sarah Lawrence College and lives with her daughter and granddaughter in New York.

**Marita Golden** is an award-winning novelist and essayist. Her books include the classic memoir *Migrations of the Heart* and the novels *Long Distance Life* and *After*. Her books are widely used in colleges and universities. She is the cofounder and president emerita of the Hurston/Wright Foundation. She has taught creative writing at George Mason University and Virginia Commonwealth University and offers her own writing workshops and literary coaching. Among her awards are the Writers for Writers Award presented by Poets & Writers and the Fiction Award presented by the Black Caucus of the ALA. Her website is www.MaritaGolden.com.

**Rebecca Newberger Goldstein**, a graduate of Barnard College who received her PhD from Princeton, is the author of ten books, of both fiction and philosophy. Her novels include *The Mind-Body Problem, Properties of Light*, and *36 Arguments for the Existence of God: A Work of Fiction*. She is also the author of *Incompleteness: The Proof and Paradox of Kurt Gödel*, named by *Discover* magazine one of the best science books of its year, and the award-winning *Betraying*

*Spinoza: The Renegade Jew Who Gave Us Modernity*. Her latest book is *Plato at the Googleplex: Why Philosophy Won't Go Away*. The recipient of numerous awards for both her fiction and her scholarship, in 1996 she was awarded a MacArthur Fellowship, popularly known as the "genius" prize. She has also been named the Humanist of the Year by the American Humanist Association and a Freethought Heroine by the Freedom from Religion Foundation. She is professor of philosophy at New College of the Humanities in London.

**Jane Green** is the author of fifteen *New York Times* best-selling novels. Initially known for writing about single thirtysomethings, Green has graduated to more complex, character-driven novels that explore the concerns of real women's lives, from relationships (*The Beach House*) to motherhood (*Another Piece of My Heart*) to divorce, stepchildren, affairs, and, most recently, midlife crises (*Family Pictures* and *Tempting Fate*). She joined the ABC News team as a writer and live correspondent covering the royal wedding, has contributed to various anthologies, and appears regularly on television shows, including *Good Morning America*, *The Martha Stewart Show*, and the *Today* show. She lives in Westport, Connecticut, with one husband, five children, two dogs, four cats, and a few chickens.

**Katie Hafner**, a native of Rochester, New York, is a frequent contributor to the *New York Times*, where she writes on health care. She has also written for the *New York Times Magazine*,

*Esquire, Wired,* the *New Republic,* the *Huffington Post,* and *O, The Oprah Magazine.* She is the author of six books of nonfiction: *Cyberpunk: Outlaws and Hackers on the Computer Frontier* (with John Markoff); *The House at the Bridge: A Story of Modern Germany; Where Wizards Stay Up Late: The Origins of the Internet* (with Matthew Lyon); *The Well: A Story of Love, Death, and Real Life in the Seminal Online Community;* and *A Romance on Three Legs: Glenn Gould's Obsessive Quest for the Perfect Piano.* Her most recent book, a memoir titled *Mother Daughter Me,* was published by Random House in 2013.

**Maria Hinojosa**'s twenty-five-year history as an award-winning journalist includes executive producing and anchoring both a radio show and television series: *Latino USA,* distributed by National Public Radio, and *America by the Numbers with Maria Hinojosa,* airing this fall on PBS and the WORLD channel. In 2010, she launched the Futuro Media Group to produce journalism giving voice to a more diverse America. Hinojosa has reported for PBS, CNN, NPR, *Frontline,* and CBS Radio and anchored the Emmy Award–winning talk show *Maria Hinojosa: One-on-One.* She is the author of two books and has won dozens of awards, including four Emmys, the John Chancellor Award, the Studs Terkel Community Media Award, the Robert F. Kennedy Award, the Edward R. Murrow Award, and the

Ruben Salazar Lifetime Achievement Award. She is currently the Sor Juana Ines de la Cruz Chair of Latin American and Latino Studies at DePaul University in Chicago and lives with her husband and their son and daughter in New York. She is a graduate of Barnard College.

**Deborah Hofmann** is a senior editor at the *New York Times*, where she oversees the best-seller lists. She has also written articles on fashion, and antiques and collectibles, as well as a wide range of general-interest profiles and feature stories, for the *Times*. She is a graduate of Barnard College and lives in Manhattan. She and her husband, Eric Asimov, are the parents of Peter and Jack.

**Siri Hustvedt** has a PhD in English literature from Columbia University. She is the author of a book of poems, *Reading to You*; three books of essays, *Mysteries of the Rectangle: Essays on Painting*, *A Plea for Eros*, and *Living, Thinking, Looking*; a work of nonfiction, *The Shaking Woman or A History of My Nerves*; and six novels: *The Blindfold*, *The Enchantment of Lily Dahl*, *What I Loved*, *The Sorrows of an American*, *The Summer Without Men*, and *The Blazing World*. *What I Loved* and *The Summer Without Men* were on the short list for the Prix Femina étranger in France. *What I Loved* won the Prix des libraires du Québec in 2003. She was the recipient of the 2012 Gabarron International Award for Thought and Humanities. Her work has been translated into over thirty languages. She lives in Brooklyn, New York.

**Suleika Jaouad** is the critically acclaimed author of the *New York Times* Well column "Life, Interrupted," which chronicles her journey as a young woman living with cancer. An award-winning video series accompanies the column, which earned Suleika a 2013 News & Documentary Emmy Award. A strong and powerful voice for the young adult generation, Suleika travels the country as a health advocate and motivational speaker.

Suleika graduated summa cum laude from Princeton University in 2010 with a BA in Near Eastern studies and a double certificate in French and women & gender studies. Shortly after graduation, at age twenty-two, Suleika was diagnosed with myelodysplastic syndrome and acute myeloid leukemia. After three years of chemotherapy and a bone marrow transplant, she is finally cancer-free and continuing to make the most of a life, interrupted.

**Deborah Jiang-Stein** is a national speaker and founder of the unPrison Project, a 501(c)3 nonprofit working to empower and inspire incarcerated women and girls with life skills and mentoring. She's the author of *Women Behind Bars: Stories from Prison* (Shebooks), a collection of interviews, and the memoir *Prison Baby* (Beacon Press).

**Emma Gilbey Keller** was born and raised in London, England. She is the author of two books, *The Lady: The Life and Times of Winnie Mandela* and *The Comeback: Seven Stories of Women Who Went from Career to Family and Back.* She has contributed to the *New York Times*, the *New Yorker*, *Vanity Fair*, the *Guardian*, and the *Daily Telegraph*, among others. She writes mainly about women for women. But she has reported on health for WNYC and frequently reviews books and items of popular culture. She lives in New York City with her husband, Bill Keller, and their two daughters, Molly and Alice.

**Anne Kreamer** is the author of *It's Always Personal: Navigating Emotion in the New Workplace* and *Going Gray: What I Learned about Beauty, Sex, Work, Motherhood, Authenticity, and Everything Else That Really Matters.* Her next book, *The Risk Factor,* is about the unprecedented professional adaptability required of everyone in the twenty-first century. Anne has also worked as a columnist for *Fast Company* and *Martha Stewart Living* and is a frequent blogger on HarvardBusinessReview.org and NextAvenue.org. Her work has appeared in *Time,* the *New York Times,* the *Wall Street Journal, Real Simple,* and *Travel + Leisure.* Previously, Anne was executive vice president and worldwide creative director for the television channels Nickelodeon and Nick at Nite. Anne graduated from Harvard College and lives in Brooklyn with her husband, the writer Kurt Andersen.

**Alex Kuczynski** is a former reporter for the *New York Times*, where she covered popular culture and the media industry. She is the author of *Beauty Junkies*, an exposé of the cosmetic surgery industry, a nonfiction book that has been translated into twelve languages. A graduate of Barnard College, she contributes to the *New York Times Book Review* and various other sections of the newspaper, and she writes for magazines. She is working on her next book.

**Anne Lamott** is the author of seven novels, including *Hard Laughter, Rosie, Joe Jones, Blue Shoe, All New People, Crooked Little Heart,* and *Imperfect Birds.* She has also written several best-selling books of nonfiction, including *Operating Instructions, Some Assembly Required: A Journal of My Son's First Son,* and *Bird by Bird: Some Instructions on Writing and Life.* Her collections of autobiographical essays on faith include *Traveling Mercies: Some Thoughts on Faith, Plan B: Further Thoughts on Faith,* and *Grace (Eventually).* Her recent books include *Help, Thanks, Wow: The Three Essential Prayers* and *Stitches: A Handbook on Meaning, Hope and Repair.*

**Honor Moore**'s most recent collection of poems is *Red Shoes.* Her memoir, *The Bishop's Daughter,* was a *New York Times* Editor's Choice, a *Los Angeles Times* favorite book of the year, and a finalist for the National Book Critics Circle Award. *The White Blackbird: A Life of the Painter Margarett Sargent by Her Granddaughter* was a *New York Times* Notable

Book. For her poetry, she has won awards from the National Endowment for the Arts and the Connecticut Commission on the Arts, and to write *The Bishop's Daughter* she was awarded a Guggenheim Fellowship. For Library of America she edited *Amy Lowell: Selected Poems* and *Poems from the Women's Movement*, an *Oprah* reading pick. A new memoir and a fourth collection of poems are forthcoming. She teaches graduate nonfiction at the New School and has been a visiting distinguished writer at Wesleyan (poetry), the University of Iowa( nonfiction), and the University of Richmond (poetry and nonfiction).

**Bharati Mukherjee** is the author of eight novels (most recently, *Miss New India, Desirable Daughters,* and *The Tree Bride*), two collections of short stories (*Darkness* and *The Middleman and Other Stories*), and numerous essays on immigration and American culture, and the coauthor, with Clark Blaise, of two books of nonfiction (*Days and Nights in Calcutta* and *The Sorrow and the Terror: The Haunting Legacy of the Air India Tragedy*). She is the first naturalized US citizen to win the National Book Critics Circle Award for Best Fiction. She is a professor emerita of English at the University of California, Berkeley.

**Rosie Schaap** is the author of the memoir *Drinking with Men,* named one of the best books of 2013 by NPR, *Library Journal,* and *BookPage.* The Drink columnist for the *New York Times Magazine* since 2011 and a contributor to *This American Life,* she has also written for *Bon Appétit, Lucky Peach, Marie Claire,* the *New York Times* Dining section, PoetryFoundation.org, *Saveur, Slate, Travel + Leisure*, and many essay anthologies. A working bartender, Schaap has previously been a fortune-teller, a librarian at a paranormal society, an editor, a preacher, a community organizer, and a manager of homeless shelters. She is currently writing a book about whiskey.

**Elizabeth Searle** is the author of four books of fiction, most recently *Girl Held in Home*, and the librettist of *Tonya & Nancy: The Rock Opera*, a show that has drawn national media attention. The rock opera, based on the Harding/Kerrigan skating scandal, has been widely performed, most recently in 2014 in Hollywood. Elizabeth's previous books are *My Body to You*, which won the Iowa Short Fiction Award; *Celebrities in Disgrace*, which was produced as a short film; and *A Four-Sided Bed*, now in development as a feature film. Her theater works have been featured on *Good Morning America*, CBS, CNN, NPR, the AP, and elsewhere. Elizabeth has had work in over a dozen anthologies, including *Don't You Forget About Me* (Simon and Schuster) and *Knitting Yarns* (Norton). She lives in Arlington, Massachusetts, with her husband and son. Her website is www .elizabethsearle.net.

**Jane Smiley**'s novel *A Thousand Acres* won the Pulitzer Prize and the National Book Critics Circle Award in 1992; her novel *The All-True Travels and Adventures of Lidie Newton* won the 1999 Spur Award for Best Novel of the West. She has been a member of the American Academy of Arts and Letters since 1987. Her novel *Horse Heaven* was short-listed for the Orange Prize in 2002, and her novel *Private Life* was chosen as one of the best books of 2010 by the *Atlantic*, the *New Yorker*, and the *Washington Post*. She has written several works of nonfiction, including *Thirteen Ways of Looking at the Novel* and *The Man Who Invented the Computer*. She has also published five volumes of a horse series for young adults, *The Horses of Oak Valley Ranch*. The third volume of Jane Smiley's trilogy, *The Last Hundred Years*, was published in 2015.

**Deborah Tannen** is university professor and professor of linguistics at Georgetown University. Among her many books, *You Just Don't Understand: Women and Men in Conversation* was on the *New York Times* best-seller list for nearly four years, including eight months as number one, and has been translated into thirty-one languages; *You're Wearing THAT?: Understanding Mothers and Daughters in Conversation* and *You Were Always Mom's Favorite!: Sisters in Conversation Throughout Their Lives* were also *New York Times* best sellers. She has written for and been featured in most major magazines and newspapers including the *New York Times*, the *Washington Post*, *USA Today*, *Time*, *Newsweek*, and the *Harvard Business Review* and has appeared on such television and radio news and information shows as *The Colbert Report*, *20/20*, *Good Morning America*,

*Oprah*, the *PBS News Hour*, *All Things Considered*, *Morning Edition*, *The Diane Rehm Show*, and many other NPR programs. Her website is www.deborahtannen.com.

**Adriana Trigiani** is beloved by millions of readers around the world for fifteen best sellers, including the blockbuster epic *The Shoemaker's Wife*; the *Big Stone Gap* series; *Lucia, Lucia*; *Rococo;* and the *Valentine* series. She is also the author of the *Viola* series for young adults and the best-selling memoir *Don't Sing at the Table*. She was an award-winning writer/producer of *The Cosby Show* and *A Different World* and showrunner and executive producer of *CityKids*. She also wrote and directed the award-winning documentary *Queens of the Big Time.*

Trigiani wrote and directed the film version of her debut novel *Big Stone Gap* for the big screen, shot entirely on location in Trigiani's hometown with an all-star cast. The film made its premiere at the Virginia Film Festival in 2014. A wife and mother, she lives in Greenwich Village with her husband, Tim Stephenson, the Emmy-winning lighting designer for *Late Show with David Letterman,* and their daughter, Lucia.

**Patricia Volk** is the author, most recently, of *Shocked: My Mother, Schiaparelli, and Me* and the memoir *Stuffed: Adventures of a Restaurant Family*. She is the author of two novels, *To My Dearest Friends* and *White Light,* and two collections of short stories. Volk is the recipient of a Guggenheim Fellowship and has taught at Columbia University, New York University, and Bennington College. Her writing has appeared in the *New York Times*, the *Atlantic*, *New York*, the *New Yorker*, and *Playboy*. She lives in New York.

# Permissions

CPSIA information can be obtained
at www.ICGtesting.com
Printed in the USA
LVOW11*1315280218
568189LV00006B/21/P